Weight Loss
WISDOM

Published by MQ Publications Limited
12 The Ivories
6-8 Northampton Street
London, N1 2HY
email: mail@mqpublications.com
website: www.mqpublications.com

Editor: Laura Kesner
Design Concept: Dennis Michael Stredney
Interior Book Design: Dennis Michael Stredney

ISBN: 1-84072-713-6

10 9 8 7 6 5 4 3 2 1

Printed and bound in China

Weight Loss
WISDOM

365 successful dieting tips

SUSIE GALVEZ

MQP

Contents

Contents

Introduction

*"I've been on a constant diet for the last two decades.
I've lost a total of 789 pounds.
By all accounts, I should be hanging from a charm bracelet."*
Erma Bombeck

Diet. **D-I-E-T**, a simple four-letter word that strikes fear and dread into the hearts of most anyone struggling to lose excess weight. However, the actual meaning of the word is quite neutral. Diet literally means: **"course of life: way of living or thinking…to regulate oneself."** *Oxford English Dictionary*

Perhaps the reason for the rather unpleasant dieting image in our mind is based on both our own experiences with weight loss and tales of woe told to us by others. Speaking from my own dieting experiences, in most cases, after everything was weighed and measured, all I usually ended up losing on a diet was my patience! Losing weight takes self-control and persistence. It also takes following a food plan that you can stick with—and actually enjoy! *Weight Loss Wisdom* is *not* a diet book. There are so many good weight-loss programs out there—you can easily find one that meets your special health or dietary needs and fits easily into your lifestyle. Finding one that works, and works safely, is not an issue. Helping you learn how to *stay* on your program is the key.

Like the famous saying *"enjoy the journey, not just the destination,"* successful long-term weight loss is more than just hitting the goal—how many times have we lost weight only to regain the amount lost, and more? *Weight Loss Wisdom* has 12 chapters brimming with ideas, tips, and techniques all designed to work with whatever weight-loss program you have chosen. You will find helpful hints on dressing slimmer, quick fixes to dieting dilemmas, great "filler up" foods, "did you know?" food facts, advice on changing recipes to fit your new lifestyle, eating out, holidays, exercising, altering your mind set, and much more!

With this book, following your weight-loss plan will be easier and your results will last. Let's get started! ♥

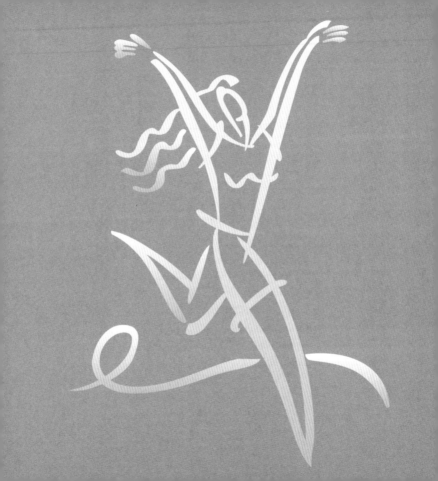

CHAPTER 1

"Surviving is important, but thriving is elegant."
Maya Angelou

Smart Thinking

Most weight-loss plans merely offer survival, and when I think of surviving I think of **"roughing it,"** not **"enjoying it."** If you put your energy into discovering ways to enjoy your weight-loss journey, I promise you that your trip will be first class all the way. **Now, read on to get your map!** ❤

Cast the MOLD

FIND A BODY-TYPE ROLE MODEL, but be
realistic so you avoid setting yourself up for
disappointment. It is like constantly picking
straight hairstyles when you have a head full of
natural curls. *Look for someone with a
body build similar to yours,* but in the
weight range that you are striving for, and model
yourself accordingly. ❤

Pay at the PUMP

Think of your body as a car and food as your fuel.

If you put high-quality food into your engine, you will perform more efficiently. If you fill your tank with low-quality, processed foods, you will feel sluggish and your body will not perform at its optimum level. ♥

Savor the Sin

Make it a rule to NEVER EAT ANYTHING THAT IS FULL OF FAT AND CALORIES IF YOU DON'T REALLY LOVE IT. Save those high calorie intakes for the foods that you are absolutely crazy about. Then eat, enjoy, and savor every last bite! ❤

Tap in on the **TAP WATER, WATER,** *and* more **WATER.**

Drinking **eight to ten** glasses of water every day will help curb your appetite, flush out waste products, and fill you up when you are hungry. *As an added bonus, your skin will look more healthy and hydrated.* This is not breaking news, but hopefully at this moment, you are on the way to fill up your glass! ♥

Change OF Pace

Instead of the "your office or mine" routine for a meeting, **try walking.** Meet in the lobby and stroll around the complex or the block while you conduct business. **The fresh air, different scenery, and the movement will get the creative juices flowing,** and you will return raring to go! ❤

Don't Drive Through

If you want it, **park it**, and go in and get it. You'll get a bit of extra exercise walking from your car, plus if it's food you are going in for, you have a few extra seconds to make a decision on exactly what you are going to get, instead of the usual grab and go. ♥

NO Deliveries

Become the courier. If you **really** are CRAVING SOMETHING, make the effort to **go and get it.** If you have to drive even ten-minutes round trip, you might just find you really don't want it after all. ❤

16

Linger **Longer**

Always **allow at least a half hour between dinner and dessert.**

You will have time to

feel full and will **most**

likely eat less. ♥

LISTEN to Your Mother

NEVER TALK WITH YOUR MOUTH FULL. Mom was right. It is also a good idea to **stop eating and listen to other people as they talk.** By doing so, both the food and the conversation will be savored. ❤

TAKE TIME *to* TAKE TIME

MAKE IT A RULE to **sit when you eat.** Eating on the run is just that. Mealtime will come and go and if you don't take the time to make time, you will scarcely remember that you ate at all. Food time needs to be penciled in your calendar, just like any other important project. ♥

19

Palm **Reader**

The size of your palm is a good measure of what a portion size should look like

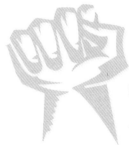

for most meats, vegetables, starchy foods, and fruit. Of course, in the candy family, it's thumbs up—use your thumb as a guide for serving size. ❤

ON *the* **A**-*List*

MAKING A GROCERY LIST BEFORE
YOU HEAD TO THE STORE WILL
HELP KEEP YOU ON TRACK AND ON
YOUR FOOD PLAN. Plus, it will no doubt
save you money, since you won't
have to guess whether you need
a particular item or not. If you
see something tempting, put it on
the list for next time. Chances are
you will be out of the mood for it
when it's time to shop again. ❤

OUT OF SIGHT

Use the fruit and vegetable bin in the refrigerator to store high-fat temptations. Chances are, you'll forget they are there. After all, **OUT OF SIGHT, OUT OF MIND,** and most importantly, **off the thighs.** ♥

22

CLEAN UP

To reduce the temptation of tasting what you are baking or cooking, **immediately put the utensils in a bowl of hot water.** By placing them in hot water straightaway, you will have less time to lick them clean. ❤

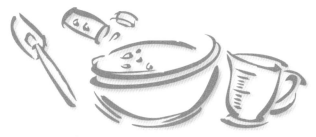

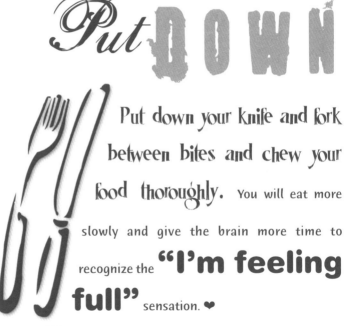

Put DOWN

Put down your knife and fork between bites and chew your food thoroughly. You will eat more slowly and give the brain more time to recognize the **"I'm feeling full"** sensation. ❤

24

WHAT'S the PASSWORD?

Change your computer password to a word or phrase that will make you **"THINK THIN"** every time you use it. How about "hourglass;" "skinny one;" "perfect size;" or think of your own trigger word. When you type it, you will think it. ♥

25

Keep It Moving FOLKS

To keep the blood and lymph flowing, TRY TO SIT NO LONGER THAN **30** MINUTES AT A TIME. If possible, stand up and walk to the water fountain or at least stand while you are on the telephone and pace back and forth. The movement is good for circulation and for food digestion. ♥

MIRROR, MIRROR
on the Wall

BUY A FULL-LENGTH MIRROR, either free-standing or one that can attach to your closet or bathroom door interior. It will show you where you want to lose weight and, as an extra bonus, you can see where you are already losing it! ❤

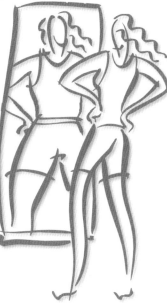

27

To the *Nines*

When dining out or spending time with friends,

wear your most flattering outfit.

You will get loads of compliments, which can be a

great reminder to watch what you put in your mouth.

Plus, it will reinforce the sense that your weight-loss program

is already working. ❤

Good Morning!

BREAKFAST is the best way to have a good morning, **and a good day!** Breakfast eaters think more creatively and work more efficiently. Plus, breakfast keeps you from grabbing the break room doughnuts—ugh! ❤

STOP and THINK

It could be just a few minutes of resting with your eyes closed that you need to restore your energy and vitality— INSTEAD OF A HIGH-CALORIE SNACK.

Try it and see for yourself. Sit with one hand cupped over each eye for 60 to 90 seconds. Block out all of the light and just breathe deeply. Open and see the world refreshed and calorie-free. ❤

MUNCHING at MIDNIGHT?

If you notice that you are munching late at night—
check your dinnertime selections.
If protein is on the skimpy
side, while carbohydrates
are in abundance, try
reversing it by increasing
the protein portion and
reducing the amount of
carbs. Protein keeps
you fuller, longer. ❤

KEEP *Convenience* Convenient

If you are a grab-it-on-the-go type of person, simply change the "grab." Opt for a protein bar instead of a candy bar, or pretzels instead of chips. The main thing is to keep the "good stuff" on hand, ready to grab and go. ♥

Pack Your BAGS

To help with portion control and save money to boot, purchase food in the larger economy size, **but right away measure out the correct serving size for your plan and put it in resealable bags or containers.** You'll be less tempted to eat the whole bagful. Plus, it is another way to streamline mealtime. ♥

Something to Chew On

Fruits and vegetables take longer to chew and eat, and as a rule, have more fiber than other food types. And since they take longer to eat, you are more likely to feel content and full. ❤

Private EYE

When questioning whether any unlabeled food is high in fat, SOMETIMES YOU CAN BE FOOLED. One sure way to tell if a food is on the fatty side is to taste a tiny bite. If the food feels thick on the tongue or gets stuck on the teeth, chances are it is a high-fat food.

Be a food sleuth. ♥

Guess
WHAT?

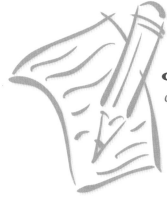

Guessing which foods are best for your weight-loss efforts is like guessing at a **MULTIPLE CHOICE QUIZ**. You are usually correct about 50 percent of the time. To increase the weight-loss odds in your favor, **pick up a pocket-size calorie counter** and keep it handy to determine which foods are best for you. ♥

BUGGY CENTRAL

To get a little extra workout while grocery shopping, **park your cart** in a less busy section of the store, like the beauty-aids aisle, and go gather what you need. By **walking back and forth to the cart,** not only will you enjoy the extra exercise, but your frustration level at not being able to maneuver the cart through the tiny aisles will vanish. ❤

GIVE it UP

Start fresh. Rid your cabinets, cupboards, and pantry shelves of all not-good-for-you foods. Give it to a charitable food pantry. A good thing to do for your spirit *and* your figure. ❤

WAIT Just a Minute

IF A SUDDEN CRAVING FOR A FATTENING FOOD HITS,
before you indulge, *run in place for two to three minutes or do 15 sit-ups or push-ups.* This burst of activity will remind you of your weight-loss goals and maybe, just maybe, the craving will fade. At the very least, you will have already worked off some of the extra calories if you do succumb to the craving! ❤

LEFT *Versus* RIGHT

If you're trying to be more conscious of your snacking habits and the amount you're eating, remember this trick. **Eat with your non-dominant hand.** If you are right-handed, use your left to dig into the popcorn. Left-handed? Use the right hand to retrieve chips from the bag. You may find that you eat less and become more aware of what you do eat. ❤

40

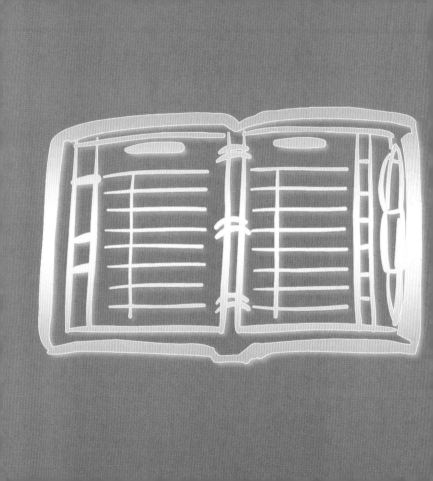

"Funny, isn't it, how your whole life goes by while you think you're only planning the way you're going to live it."
Edna Ferber

Slimming Strategies

H aving a strategic plan in any business is critical for its success. *You are in the business of successful long-term weight loss.* However, having a plan and actually following it are two different things. Make a pact right here and now to add some of the slimming strategies that you will learn in this chapter to your to-do list, **and start doing them today!** ❤

TWO Will Do

When bread is included in a meal, **keep the serving to two ounces.** Each slice of bread is about one ounce, and a dinner roll averages two ounces. Half a bagel is between one and one-half to two ounces.

Include this *"staff of life"* in your daily plans, but don't overindulge. ❤

Wake-Up Call

If breakfast is not your "cup of tea," spread it out. Break it up by dividing it into two snacks—**one for the morning, and the other for the afternoon**, when most cravings hit. Take whatever is usually suggested on your meal plan, divide it in two, and you are all set. ❤

Club *200*

A healthy snack or mini-meal replacement consists of **200** calories. In a pinch, do you know what low-calorie food you could grab on the go? If so, good for you. If not, right here and now, pre-plan some **200**-calorie selections.

Suggestions:

a meal-replacement bar or shake; **a boiled egg and slice of toast;** *a piece of fruit and a serving of* yogurt or cottage cheese; *or perhaps a garden salad with a mozzarella cheese stick*. Think of other foods that will work for you, so you will always be prepared to stay on plan. ❤

46

Know Your **A**-**B**-**C**s

If your food plan does not have column A, column B,
and column C selection suggestions, make your own.
Column A could be protein sources with a range
of 150 to 200 calories. **Column B** is starch;
column C is vegetables; **column D** is fruit; and
finally, **column E** is fats/oils. Make a grid and keep
it handy. Simply pick one from each category based
on your needs. This will help you put together great,
nutritionally sound meals. ❤

TRADE IN

Eating planned snacks on smaller plates, such as a **salad plate** or **dessert plate**, instead of a dinner plate, will help to make the serving look bigger. A sliced-up piece of fruit and a scoop of cottage cheese, surrounded by a few crackers, will make an array of eating pleasure, and you will feel like you have had more than you did. ❤

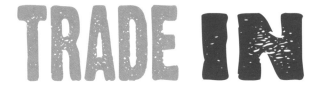

Close SHAVE

Once or twice a week, **eat 250 calories less than your weight-loss program requires.** You will be amazed at how easily this can be accomplished. Forgo the extra one-half cup of breakfast cereal here, or the pat of butter off the potato or rice there. Maybe choose a *lower calorie entrée.* Believe it or not, **twice a week X 250 X 52** weeks for the year **equals 12 to 15 pounds** shaved off! ❤

"My Other Body Is..."

Like the bumper stickers that say "my other car is a Rolls-Royce," come up with your own slogan that fits where you want to be. Maybe "my other body is a size ten" or "my other body is fit and healthy."

Cut out photos of clothes and people who have the body style you are seeking and create a storyboard that reflects your goal. Keep it somewhere prominent and look at it daily. ❤

weekend **watch**

Although exercising throughout the week is the ideal, weekends usually offer more leisure time in which to increase your activity levels. **At least plan on walking, biking, or the like, on these two days of the week.** You will feel better, firmer, and more in control of your destiny. ❤

Switch IT

If you are often mindlessly eating foods such as fattening sweets or extra portions of cheese— **STOP AND THINK.** Instead of continuing on this downward spiral, switch the sweets for tomato slices or a bite of green onion. Replace foods such as cheeses and other savory bites with a mouthful of banana or watermelon. The switch will startle your taste buds and signal the brain to regain control. ♥

CUPBOARD *Keepers*

To ensure a successful weight-loss journey, keep healthy,
easy-to-prepare items, such as whole-wheat pasta,
couscous, or brown rice, along with canned
tomato products, such as diced tomatoes with
extra spices, or tomato sauce, on hand for a
quick meal. Add some vegetables and you
have a healthy meal at your fingertips! ❤

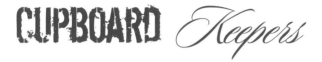

+ DO THE MATH

Walking slowly burns an average of five calories a minute. Pick up the pace to more brisk treks and step up the calories burned to ten per minute. Let's see, 30 minutes at a quick pace equals 300 calories burned. **Hmmmm,** times five days a week, times 52 weeks a year equals 78,000 calories, divided by 3,500 (the number of burned calories needed to lose one pound) equals 1.85 pounds a month and 22.29 pounds per year. Totals tell. Get up and start moving. While you walk, think about how smart you are to figure all this out! ❤

54

Green GIANT

Green salads are one of the healthiest foods you can consume.

No fat, and high in fiber and nutrients. This tasty addition needs to be included in both your lunch and dinner meals as often as possible. Studies show that eating two salads saves up to 350 calories a day. This is due to the volume that salads provide, filling you up, and lessening the want for other foods. It doesn't take long to measure those savings. ♥

55

Kitchen Radar

Periodically **"radar"** your kitchen for **foods that are not good for you**, but have somehow made it back into the cupboard, cabinet, or fridge. Take a look at the invaders and decide what to keep for weight-loss success, and what to toss or donate to the office snack table. **You will be amazed at what bad-for-you food aliens lurk in the average kitchen.** ♥

Muffin Menace

A so-called healthy muffin can still pack some scary statistics.

Fat-free versions can be the most deceiving. Instead of fat, sugar is added by the spoonful. Even a really **"healthy"** muffin can contain 400 calories! Add that to morning fruit and a cup of yogurt and the total is out of the ballpark. Recent studies show a **"healthy"** 400-calorie muffin, five days a week equals 104,000 calories or 29 pounds a year. Think about all of the 200-calorie morning alternatives and smile at the 15-pounds-a-year savings! ♥

Don't Sweat It

Sweat clothes are comfortable and relaxing, but don't fall into the fat trap. **Hiding under oversized sweats or cotton clothes is comforting, but can lead to denial.** Baggy, ill-fitting outfits allow us to forget about body silhouettes. Wearing more form-fitting garments increases body awareness and weight-loss success. Keep sweats true to size and toss the too big, extra-portion kind. ♥

HELP WANTED

The old saying "the more you give, the more you get" is true for weight loss too. **Find a diet buddy** and share ideas and successes. **Listen, Really Listen to Her Situation and Offer Solutions.** Allow her to suggest ways in which to help you succeed. You will be doing a good deed for her and helping yourself along the way. ❤

Perfect Pampering

Pamper yourself. Remember, you are a unique individual and worth every penny. **Make an appointment for a facial, massage, pedicure, manicure, or all of the above.**

Make a date to treat yourself to a bubble bath. Find a good book, light some candles in the bathroom, close the door, and really enjoy your "me time." ❤

Life Commitment

The facts speak for themselves. People who have meaning in their lives, something that gives them purpose and drive, are healthier. *Find the thing that gives you purpose,* be it a fulfilling career, community involvement, religious work—anything that makes you feel positive about yourself and allows you to *live with more passion and happiness.* This positive outlook will help you stick to your weight-loss program. ❤

DON'T *Quit* NOW

If the task of dieting is overwhelming right this minute, **decide to quit—later.**

Give yourself just one more day on your diet. Chances are that the urge to continue and win will spur you on to the glory of victory, instead of the agony of defeat. ❤

Count on Carbs

Carbohydrates, while given poor press in recent years, are still the best way to get the most nutrients without the fat. **Whole-wheat pasta, brown rice, and sweet potatoes are all good for any weight-loss plan,** provided they are accounted for and eaten in proper portions. Additionally, since such foods are palate-pleasers, you will feel satisfied, not deprived. ❤

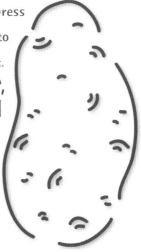

PERSON *Seeking* Person

To see how you sell yourself, write an imaginary personal ad for yourself, focusing first on your physical characteristics. What word would you use—voluptuous, statuesque, Rubenesque, or another adjective? What about your inner self, your likes and desires? Review your ad. Is this a person you would like to know? If so, great! If not, all the more reason to stick to your weight-loss plan. ❤

TRIGGER Happy

Learn to avoid anti-weight-loss "TRIGGERS" or weight-loss saboteurs.

If family gatherings or happy hours send your weight-loss plan out the door, decide how to handle these situations or avoid them for a while. Bow out until you feel more confident and in control. If having a certain food in the house is a dangerous temptation, remove the food. Opt instead to have plenty of healthy foods at home that you can eat at a moment's notice. While it is impossible to avoid everything that sabotages your diet plan, at least you can minimize the choices. ♥

Sign Me UP

Sign on for the long term.

Adopt a healthier lifestyle for a lifetime, not just to achieve a weight-loss goal. When you replace poor habits with good, you are securing the way to keeping the weight off. Remember, eating right, exercising, and taking care of yourself is a lifestyle decision. *The benefits are lifelong.* ❤

SUM it UP

If you haven't already got one, invest in a pocket-size calorie counter book. Use the book regularly, so you can learn the caloric content for a variety of foods. With this knowledge at your fingertips, you will definitely advance to the head of the math class. To say nothing of the weight-loss class! ♥

CALORIES

Make the COMMITMENT

Weight-loss plans that focus only on losing weight will not be helpful at teaching you how to keep the weight off. To be most effective, **the ideal plan will focus both on losing weight and maintaining the weight loss.** The best plans will offer ideas for meal planning and healthy eating. Before deciding which plan to follow, thoroughly research your options and gain an understanding of how a particular program will fit into your lifestyle for the longterm. ❤

PEP Talk

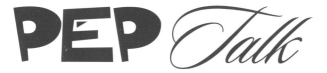

Rally around to get ready for the long haul. There's no doubt that getting ready psychologically is critical to long-term weight loss. You already know that you want/need to lose weight; how much you need to lose; and that a good food plan is important to getting you there. Now the final step is to psych yourself up to make it happen. **RAH! RAH! RAH! RIGHT! LOSE 'EM UP, WAY UP!** ♥

Make it a MYSTERY

If you have friends or family members who are skeptical of your weight-loss plans—or who seem to delight when you fail to achieve your goals—**KEEP YOUR PLANS TO YOURSELF.** Let them be pleasantly surprised by your success, and maybe even a little jealous of your progress. ♥

70

RENEW Your Contract

Remember why you decided to lose weight in the first place—remind yourself of your initial goals to help you keep track. Your contract can be reviewed and renewed. Make any changes you need to be successful. ♥

READ All About It

Keep up with what's what in the weight-loss world. While the goal is not to jump from diet to diet, it's good to know the latest information. The most

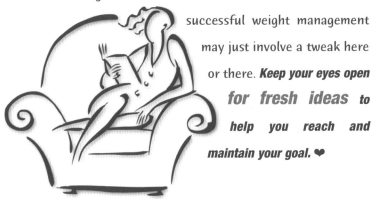

successful weight management may just involve a tweak here or there. **Keep your eyes open for fresh ideas to help you reach and maintain your goal.** ❤

Beginner's **LUCK**

A recent university study concluded that **we are most likely to lose weight on a diet if we haven't tried that particular diet in the past.** This could be because we often respond positively to novelty. Second, we have to pay closer attention in order to learn the new program, but with a previously tried program, we have figured out all of the ins and outs and find it easy to take shortcuts. ❤

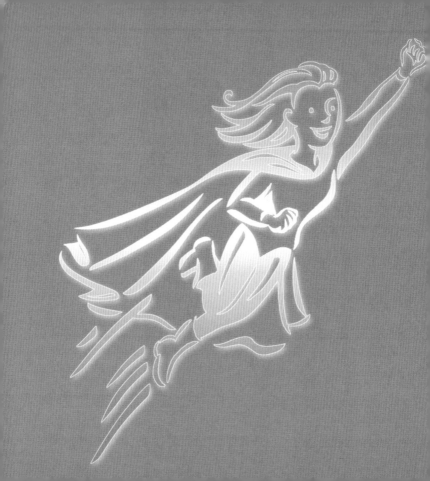

"There are so many things that we wish we had done yesterday,
so few that we feel like doing today."
Mignon McLaughlin

Quick Fixes

While there is no magic pill to cure our weight-loss woes overnight, there are quick and easy fixes to most any weight-loss dilemma. Whether you're experiencing water retention, an afternoon energy slump, or the "uh-oh, I should *not* have eaten that" blues, this chapter will arm you with the fight-fat-back knowledge that you need to *emerge victorious from your weight-loss battle.* ❤

BOWLED OVER

MAKE A BIG, FRESH, GREEN SALAD AND KEEP IT IN A LARGE, SEALED BOWL IN THE REFRIGERATOR. Perfect for on the run, quick fixes in the veggie department. *You can easily take out a serving at a time,* so packing lunches is a snap! ❤

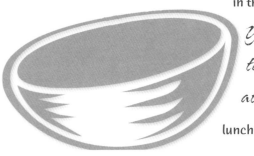

SHOW and TELL

If you have lost weight, but have hit a plateau, go to the grocery store and pick up what you have lost. Whether it's a **five-pound** bag of sugar, a **ten-pound** sack of potatoes, or **15 pounds** of kitty litter, you will realize what an amazing feat you have already accomplished. *Feeling the weight in your hands and knowing that it was once on you, puts the plateau in perspective.* ♥

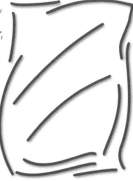

OUT with the OLD

As you shed the weight, shed the clothes. *Box up and give to charity all of your,* **now too big for you,** *clothes.* You will need the room for all of your new slim-outfits. If you simply cannot part with them, loan them to a friend who is your former size. At least you'll be able to occasionally visit with your old clothes. ❤

Breath of FRESH AIR

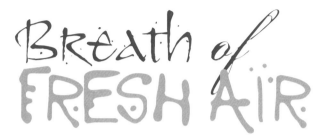

BREATH MINTS ARE GREAT TO KEEP HANDY.

At less than five calories each, they freshen your

breath and, just maybe,

lessen the allure of that

tempting treat. **Pop a**

mint instead. ♥

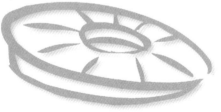

Mug SHOT

FLAVORED COFFEES CAN GIVE YOU A RICH TASTE AND A FULL FEELING DURING THE DAY, *without the calories.*

A cup of bouillon broth also works great. Keep some cubes in your desk drawer or briefcase for that perfect anytime pick-me-up. ❤

If You Are Stuck—DEDUCT

If the scale is not moving, **try limiting carbohydrates to only two servings a day, for a few days.** Best foods to choose from are brown rice, sweet potatoes, whole-grain bread, or whole-wheat pasta. The scale arrow should once again point south, in little or no time. ❤

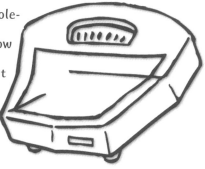

FORGO THE FIZZ

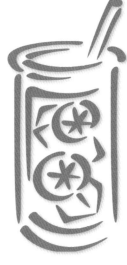

If you feel bloated—waistlines are suddenly a little snug or rings a bit tight—try eliminating carbonated beverages. **Drink flavored water, or spring water, with a squeeze of lime or lemon instead.** The extra water's good for you anyway! ❤

FOUR O'CLOCK
FORTRESS

To fend off the **FOUR O'CLOCK HUNGER SLUMP, try eating an apple with a cup of herbal tea.** The fiber of the apple will fill you up, while the herbal tea will soothe and satisfy. ❤

Staff of Life

When other craving remedies fail, **eating a single slice of multi-grain bread, very slowly, can stop a full-blown crave attack before it starts.** The trick is to eat very slowly and only eat one slice. The slice is less than 60 calories, if you choose the light variety, and totally worth it if you stop the craving in its tracks. ❤

BLOAT Be Gone

Eating bananas, broccoli, spinach, kale, or melon, especially before and during a monthly cycle

will help rid the body of excess water. Plan to add some of these water-shedding foods to your diet during "that time of the month"—you know the one! ❤

GET OVER IT

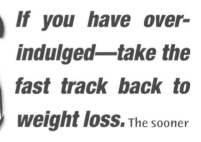

If you have over-indulged—take the fast track back to weight loss. The sooner you get back on track, the easier it will be to get over the setback. Remember it's over, so get over it. ♥

MORNING *Milk*

If you are finding it impossible to consume your calcium serving in the form of a glass of skim milk— *try and drink your morning latte with skim milk,* or pour it over your breakfast cereal. All the goodness and far fewer calories.❤

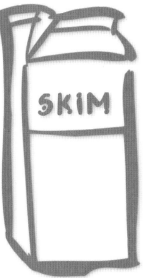

What's That Noise?

To banish those AFTERNOON STOMACH NOISES,

reach for a healthy energy bar. Best

choices will have at least 15 grams of protein.

The bar will ease the hunger pangs and help fortify

you with "anti-craving" feelings until your next

scheduled meal. ❤

DARK VICTORY

When given a choice, opt for **DARK CHOCOLATE** instead of the milk chocolate variety. A full ounce of dark chocolate contains about 110 calories—far fewer calories than in milk chocolate. But the sinfully rich, full flavor will feel and taste so much better than the run-of-the-mill milk chocolate variety. ♥

Combined EFFORTS

For a quick pick-me-up, give yourself a mini-facial, ending with a deep treatment facial mask. While the mask is working, do some reps with dumbbells and a few knee bends. The exercise will have your blood pumping and, as a bonus, your skin will benefit from the increased circulation and the hydrating effects of the mask. ❤

Bye-Bye FAT

To reduce the fat in ground beef, brown it and wait before cooking it any further. **After browning, place beef in a colander and rinse with very hot water.** The fat will be flushed down the drain. ❤

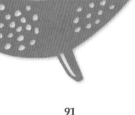

DRAT that DAB

A little DAB could do you in.

The calorie content of a lick off the spoon here, and a finger to clean off the knife there may surprise you. One tablespoon of *cake icing* is hovering at about 60 calories; *peanut butter* packs about 100 calories for that knife-full; and one tablespoon of *cream cheese* is at least 50 calories. A tablespoon of *sour cream* weighs in at 50 or so calories. So you see, *"cleaning up"* is really "counting up." ♥

Water SPORTS

If getting your recommended daily water intake is just too hard, **s p r e a d   i t   o u t.** Fill up your coffee mug with water at least twice after you have finished your morning coffee. Carry a sports bottle (20-plus ounces) to work and consume throughout the day. Then keep another bottle ready to sip on while changing clothes, preparing dinner, etc. Before you know it, your water requirements will have been met! ♥

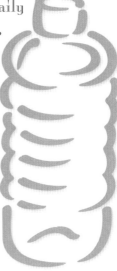

Instant *Appeal*

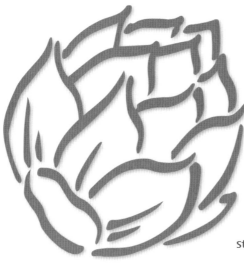

For a rich flavor with hardly any calories, USE MARINATED ARTICHOKE HEARTS IN DIFFERENT DISHES. Great for sprinkling on pizza, adding to salads, or eating as an appetizer. Save the marinade to add to vegetables, stir into pasta, or even marinate meat before grilling. ♥

94

Sundae TREAT

If an old-fashioned sundae **is what you simply must have, then sundaes it will be.** Use one-half cup of frozen yogurt, some slices of banana, peach, and strawberry (a few of each) and top with one tablespoon of chocolate syrup. Believe it or not, the chocolate syrup only has about 50 calories, the frozen yogurt (read the label) about 100, and the fruit slices weigh in at 50 to 60 calories. All together a sweet dessert with only about 200 calories. Planned-for treats add to life's satisfaction without adding to the waistline. *(Remember, the key word is "planned.")* ♥

READY and *Waiting*

Not much time to peel, slice, and prep? Do it all at one time—once a week. Visit the grocer's fresh vegetable section and pick up some **fresh greens**—green beans, squash, carrots, or any other of your favorite veggies and cut, slice, and/or grate them. Place in sealable plastic bags and keep in the least light-exposed part of the refrigerator. *Now you will have fresh, ready-to-go, vegetables to select from for your meals*—and all of the work is done! ❤

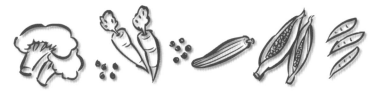

BATCH it, Freeze It, Heat n' Enjoy

Once or twice a month make meals ahead of time. Put into proper portion size, and **freeze for quick meals without the fuss.** You might not be so tempted to pull into the fast food drive-thru, if you know that you have a dish such as chicken picante with veggies waiting for you at home. ❤

The Magic Way DOES NOT EXIST

If a quick fix to weight loss is what you are seeking, KEEP SEARCHING. There are two-day, three-day, and five-day diets that you can drink, chew, or swallow. Sure, you may lose a pound a day—for a while. But as soon as normal eating is resumed, so is the weight. Opt instead for a slow and steady pace—the long-term, permanent way to lose and keep off weight. Remember, if it is fast, chances are it wont last! ♥

Substitute Teacher

Study ways to substitute lower-fat, lower-calorie, healthier foods for high-fat/high-calorie options.

For example, sour cream is **50**-plus calories a tablespoon, while plain, low-fat yogurt has only **ten.** Regular mayonnaise is over **100** calories a serving, while mustard adds only **five** calories to your sandwich. Think about ways to jazz up your dishes with the minimal amount of calories. ❤

My Compliments to the Chef

If your idea of seasoning is salt and pepper— **allow me to introduce you to a world of sauces, seasonings, and flavorings.** Fresh or dried herbs and spices, flavored vinegars, mustard spreads, light soy sauce, marinades of fruit, and meat rubs, will not only add zest to your food, but introduce you to a whole, new range of calorie-free flavors. Your taste buds will thank you. ❤

100

Insurance POLICY

Pre-planning meals is *good* *insurance* against a free-fall food fest. If you have planned your meals for the week, prepared the necessary ingredients, maybe even pre-made the entrées, you are all set, and worthy of a double indemnity policy. ❤

Home Plate

WHEN EATING AT HOME, PUT ALL OF THE FOOD ON YOUR PLATE.

Never, never, never, eat anything out of a bag, a pot, or the oven. You will be amazed at your progress if you always run first to home plate! ❤

Pleasant Dreams

When temptation is knocking on the door, think about how much better you will feel at your ideal weight. Dream about the clothes you'll wear, the way you will feel, the admiring glances you will receive, to say nothing about the confidence you will exude. Will the satisfaction you get from the food/drink you are thinking of consuming be as fulfilling? The future is now. ❤

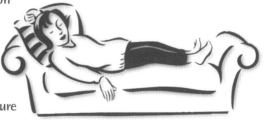

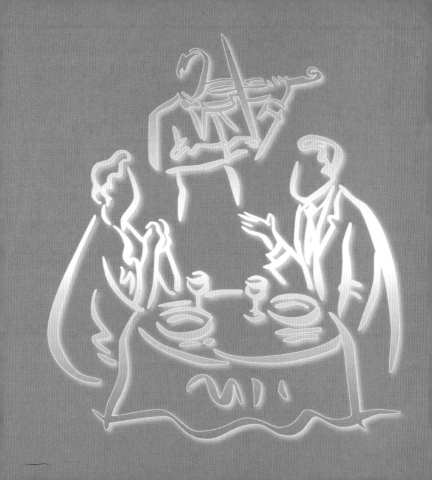

4

"If we take care of the moments, the years will take care of themselves."
Maria Edgeworth

Out and About

Dining out does not have to be a DIETING DISASTER. In fact, with proper planning, you can confidently apply the tips from this chapter and find that success while eating out is the **entrée du jour.** ❤

105

Can We SHARE?

When dining out with someone, **decide on an entrée that you can share** *and order an extra salad.* Not only is it less expensive, but you will also reduce your calorie intake by half and for once, will not leave the restaurant overstuffed. ♥

What's Nouvelle with You?

Next time you have the opportunity to dine out, why not try the newest trendy restaurant in town?

Chances are the food will be beautifully prepared and fancily presented. The artful touches and fresh herbs are not only appealing to the eye, but they also take up space on the plate! ❤

On the Road Again

Pack a cooler with some snacks, and a chilled meal or two to take with you while traveling. Not only will you feel more in control, but knowing that what you've eaten was healthy and in line with your goals is a powerful motivator for the rest of your trip. ❤

Fly the FRIENDLY SKIES

When purchasing an airline ticket, request a special meal such as low-fat, low-calorie, or the vegetarian option. Not only will your meal look and taste better than regular airline food, since you ordered a special meal, you will be served first. ❤

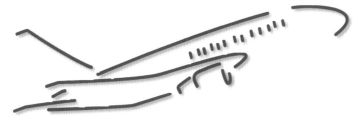

Take Two *to Go*

If your hotel has a breakfast buffet, *take a couple of extra pieces of fruit and maybe a granola bar as you leave.* This way you will have a fresh and healthy evening snack in your room, instead of staring at the vending-machine options. ♥

JUST *Desserts*

When the dessert cart rolls around, see if your

dining companion would agree to share a dessert.

Even better if you are in a group and every-

one agrees to **share that one**

'TO DIE FOR'

sweet indulgence.

Sweet on the lips without

forever on the hips. ♥

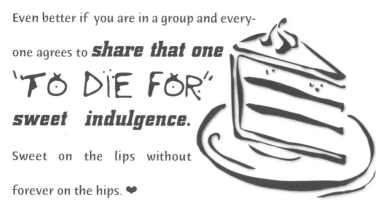

Just *the fax*

Before going to a new restaurant, **have the menu faxed or e-mailed to you.** This will allow time to see what the choices are and to make your low-calorie choice before you arrive at the restaurant—without the waiter staring at you while you stare at the menu. ♥

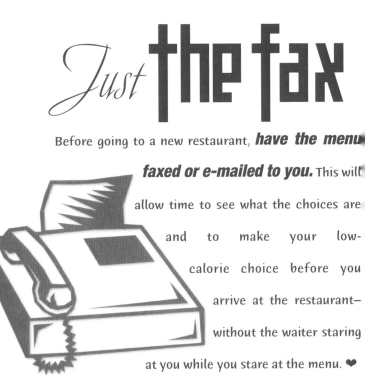

ON Foot

While vacationing, **see if your destination offers walking tours.** Walking will allow you to experience much more of the culture and uniqueness of the area than a tour bus will. To say nothing of the excellent exercise benefits. ♥

H_2O to Go

Whether traveling by land, sea, or air, **KEEP HYDRATED AND ENJOY A FULL FEELING BY DRINKING PLENTY OF WATER** and making sure you always have a bottle to hand. ❤

114

TAKE THE EDGE OFF EATING

Eating a good-for-you snack before leaving for a restaurant just might help ward off the temptation of the breadbasket. With your hunger eased, you will be able to make smart and healthy meal choices. ❤

Imbibe in Style

If you plan on having a cocktail before dinner, decide to indulge in an expensive drink such as a very good wine or a delicious martini.

You will find that you savor the higher-priced drink and thus drink less. Calories will be saved and savoir faire enhanced. ❤

Take the *Edge Off*

As soon as you sit down in a restaurant, ask for a large glass of water with a slice of lemon or lime. Drink the entire glass before you order your meal. The water will help supply a feeling of fullness, so by the time the entrée arrives, the famished feeling is gone. ❤

It's a
STRETCH

Exercise bands, also known as resistance bands, **are perfect to pack in a suitcase.** In your hotel room, you can get some resistance exercise done while on the telephone or watching TV. ❤

118

Give Me **FIVE**

Get in the habit of racing the clock to find a low-fat, low-calorie entrée on the menu. Stop when you see it, order it, and close the menu. *Chances are, the longer you look at the menu, the more tempted by less healthy choices you will become.* ♥

The Deep

More dieters are afraid of the beach than of any other travel destination. *It is not because of the sharks—***but the swimsuit!** Now, thanks to modern technology, the swimsuit is no longer anything to fear. Look for suits with underwire, tummy support panels, and a high spandex content. These waist-whittling, bust-enhancing, cellulite-smoothing garments are state-of-the-art. Ask about a matching cover-up for those moonlit strolls along the water's edge. ❤

COOKING Caution

use caution when ordering grilled vegetables while dining out. In most cases, the vegetables have been coated with oil or butter. Vegetables with softer consistencies, such as squash, eggplant, and tomatoes fare the worst. The oil or butter is absorbed like a sponge.

Ask instead for steamed vegetables whenever possible. ♥

Cuisine *Cruising*

Instead of dining on the same-old same-old, *why not try a different cuisine each time?* It could be Indian one time, Japanese the next, then Thai, and on and on. By trying new dishes, you are more likely to study the menu for the healthy choices, plus, you get to enjoy something out of the ordinary. ❤

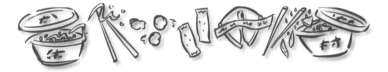

LocalFARE

While you travel, plan on enjoying local fare. **Taste the local favorite, whatever it is.** Don't worry about the calories—the extra walking and sightseeing will more than make up for any extra calories. And you will take home wonderful memories of how you enjoyed and really savored the country inside and out. ♥

Now and Later

1/2

In a restaurant, order an entrée and ask to be served **one half now and the other half wrapped up to take home.** That way, you are less likely to keep nibbling while you are not even hungry, and you have a meal ready for tomorrow. ❤

Glide ON

For a fun outing and mini-sightseeing tour, **rent a pair of inline skates and protective gear.** Glide around the town. Great exercise and you never know who you will run into!

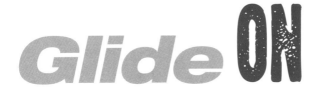

Start the Day WITH A **PLAN**

If your plans call for a meal out, embrace the calories rather than be surprised by them. Think about what you might have so you can stay **ahead of the weight-loss game.** That

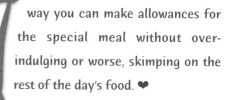

way you can make allowances for the special meal without over-indulging or worse, skimping on the rest of the day's food. ❤

ALMOST half way

Currently, **ALMOST HALF** *of all money spent on food is eaten outside the home.* Whether due to hectic work schedules, or simply being too tired to cook, eating out is now the norm. So just remembering to be healthy when eating at home is only half of the battle. **LEARNING TO MAKE SENSIBLE CHOICES WHILE ENJOYING A MEAL OUT IS CRITICAL TO ANY WEIGHT-LOSS SUCCESS.** ❤

Speak UP

Just because the menu says fried, doesn't mean it has to be. **Ask for the food to be baked, grilled, or broiled instead.** You will save **ten to 40** grams of fat and about **300** calories per entrée. Also, ask for salsa rather than butter for your baked potato. If the waitperson balks, tell them you are allergic to fat—when you eat it, you break out. ♥

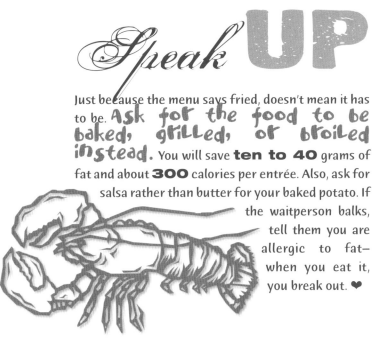

Go Pro

If travel plans permit, **take a lesson with a golf or tennis pro at a nice resort.** Even if you are not staying as a guest, most resorts offer lessons to day visitors. You'll be mingling with the jet set and getting some extra exercise. ❤

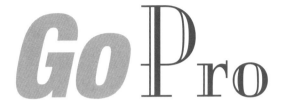

Divide and
Conquer

Your dinner entrée should consist of **50 percent** vegetables, **25 percent** meat, and **25 percent** starch. If the entrée does not seem to add up, add an extra portion of vegetables or cut your meat and starch in half and ask the wait staff to box it up so you can take it home. ❤

Pick **TWO** Out of **THREE**

When it comes to bread, desserts, and alcohol, all of which are unnecessary food choices, **make it a rule to pick two out of the three.** That way you will feel in control.

Uhmmm, what will it be? The wine and cheesecake or the bread and the flan? **SUCH CHOICES!** ❤

Vacation Indulgence

Designate one meal a day as your indulgence meal.

If you simply must have the bread, cheese, olive oil, 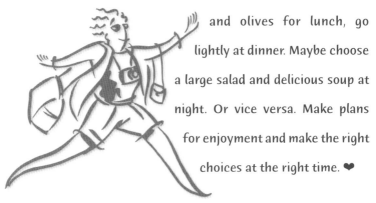 and olives for lunch, go lightly at dinner. Maybe choose a large salad and delicious soup at night. Or vice versa. Make plans for enjoyment and make the right choices at the right time. ❤

Freeze FRAME

When travel plans keep you gone too long to have fresh food waiting for your return, freeze it. **Have plenty of good-for-you foods in the freezer**—especially for the first one or two days after your trip, until you can shop for fresh. ❤

A DIFFERENT MODE
of Transportation

When traveling, see the sights on a tandem bike, paddleboat, or canoe, with someone special

You will have a vacation to remember and most likely no weight gain. ♥

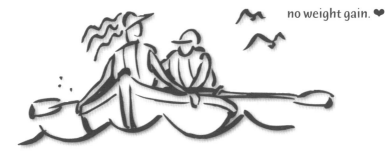

Stash a Snack

To keep temptation far, far away, **keep an easy-to-stash snack in your purse, your briefcase, or your backpack.** You will have a healthy, good-for-you, snack at arms length for times when those meetings lag on, and on. Or when running a few errands turns into an all day shopping excursion. Or when you discover that there is a two-hour wait for a table! ❤

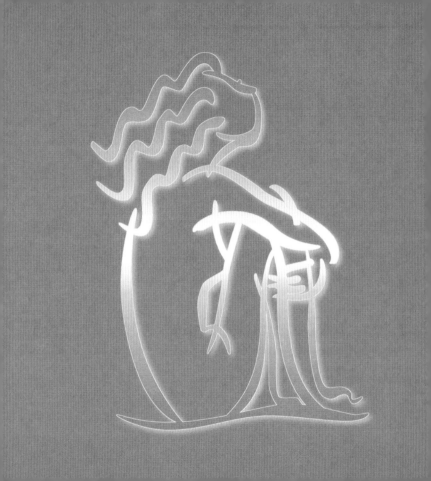

CHAPTER 5

"Can't nothin' make your life work if you ain't the architect."
Terry McMillan

Mind Games

Mind over matter really is the key when it comes to realizing your dreams. This chapter will teach you how to perceive your body in new ways, *which in turn, will change the way you think about weight loss, forever.* ❤

137

Get REAL

Be forgiving and be realistic. **celebrate the small victories.** Remember, this is not an all-or-nothing proposition. This is life. Some days will be filled with excellent choices for food and exercise, while others will be full of challenges and questionable choices. **DON'T LET YOURSELF GET DISCOURAGED. Remember, you've come a long way.** ♥

OUT OF *This World*

No foods are on a path to extinction. **Rest assured that anything you have decided to temporarily give up** for the cause (because it is not helping you to achieve your goals) **will still be on earth once you have reached your goal.** ♥

Mirror, Mirror

Take the mirror test. Look at yourself and describe out loud what you see. Look at and feel all of the curves you rarely notice or choose to ignore; study the areas you are pleased with and feel positive about. **Make a commitment to change anything you think needs work.** And please, allow yourself to accept a compliment from yourself because you are your own unique being. ❤

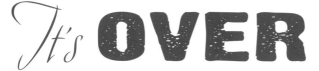

It's **OVER**

As soon as you have finished eating, remove your

plate from the table. If dining out, cover your plate

with your napkin. **This will signal**

to the brain that the

meal is over. ♥

A PICTURE
is worth a thousand words

If you have one, put a picture of you at your dream weight, or at your largest on the refrigerator. The photo will inspire you, one way or another.

If you have an extra photo, keep it on your bathroom mirror. ❤

Take a Hike

If a sudden food craving hits, *go for a brisk walk.* Think about how good it feels to have the willpower to overcome the temptation, and be proud of yourself! ♥

FLIP *the Switch*

While dining, turn off the TV and play some soft instrumental music in the background. It will add enjoyment to your meals and will also help slow the eating pace, therefore aiding digestion. ❤

REDEFiNED

Take a look at your relationship with food. **See what role it plays in your daily life. Is it for** *comfort?* STRESS? BOREDOM? Food in its proper place supplies nourishment and energy. Eating for other reasons may need to be addressed. ❤

Silence is Golden

LIMITING TALK WHILE YOU EAT, *especially while at work,* **WILL HELP YOU TO FEEL MORE SATISFIED WITH YOUR MEAL.** Excessive talking can keep you from being aware of your food, and you may just "wolf it down" before you realize you've even eaten. Talk less, eat more slowly, and feel fuller for longer. ❤

146

Go FOR THE GOAL

Setting realistic goals for yourself gives you a timeline to follow. *Losing ten pounds in 90 days;* being at your ideal weight this time next year; exercising three times a week, and the like, are promises to make to yourself. Remember the key words, **"Be realistic."** ♥

MATCH *Your Mood*

If you simply have to give in to your craving, **match the food to your mood.** Feeling stressed? Go for crunchy pretzels, pita chips, or vegetables. Need comforting? Low-fat pudding or sugar-free gelatin with a spoon of whipped cream could be just the ticket. ❤

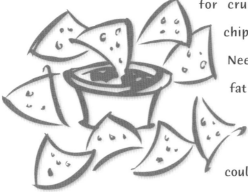

148

FAT *versus* SLIM

LIST THE TOP FIVE REASONS WHY YOU DON'T WANT TO BE FAT. Then jot down your top five answers to why slim is better. See them in black and white. Keep your lists where you can see them daily. ❤

Make It count

Every bite you eat counts in the scheme of things.

Choose foods that confirm your success. Skip the

foods that counteract your goal. I bet you know

which foods are which! ❤

Savor the Moment

Enjoy your meals, love what you eat, and eat the foods that you know are good for you. Slow down and taste the delicious life-affirming nutrients in each bite. ♥

MMMMMMMMMM!

To **WEIGH** or Not to **WEIGH**?
THAT IS THE QUESTION.

If you find it better to weigh yourself each morning to keep things in check, then do so. If weighing is only going to disappoint and set you up to fail, then

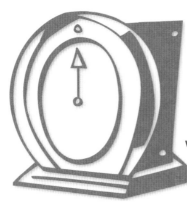

don't do it. Hopping on the scale more than once a day is not advisable under any circumstances. Food, fluids, clothing, shoes, etc. will always affect the scale and thus your state of mind. ♥

THREE DAYS *Tops*

That is the longest amount of time that it could take you to recoup after overindulging, so don't fret, you haven't blown it—unless you continue down that path. Get back on track immediately. **Next time you might even ask yourself ahead of time if three days' extra deprivation is worth the splurge.** Mmmmm…good question, don't you think? ❤

Scarlett SAID IT

"*After all, tomorrow is another day.*"

Each day is fresh, new, and waiting to be lived.

It is **24** hours in which you can enjoy and

relish your healthy habits. Live your life plan one day

at a time. ♥

154

CHA, CHA, CHANGES

changes are a part of life. Remember, if you are not

changing for the better, you are changing for the

worse. What three steps can you take that will make

a change for the better in your life today? ❤

Thoughts to PONDER

Understanding why you do what you do is critical to your success.

Take a look at your food plan, your exercise program, and your long-range goals. Are you meeting them? Are they satisfying? Can they keep you on track for success? If so, great. Continue with your plan. If not, stop and reevaluate what is missing or not working and make adjustments. ❤

THINK THIN

Being thin is as much a result of thinking thin as it is of eating the right foods. Planning the way to be thin, eating the right foods, and doing the right exercises are only part of the battle. MENTALLY, LET GO OF YOUR FORMER FAT SELF AND DISCOVER THE thin PERSON DESPERATE TO GET OUT. ❤

Accept the EXCEPTIONS

FACE it, SOME DAYS ARE JUST PLAIN BETTER THAN OTHERS.

Dinners out with no choices, the catered all-day business meeting, the social gathering with limited and mostly fattening choices, are all present, real challenges to even the most disciplined dieter's regimen. Life happens. **Learn to make the exception exceptional!**

Instead of worrying about what you ate, concentrate on how you remove those extra calories and fat from the body as effortlessly as you added them! ♥

GET IT, GOT IT, *Live it*

BELIEVE IT OR NOT, getting thin is much easier than staying thin. For the most part, portions and choices while on a weight-loss program are predetermined, so when you're finished, you're finished. Maintenance, however, is a bit trickier. Foods and/or portions, which were restricted or limited, now have to be reintroduced into your "civilian" life. **Remember to take it slow.** What difference will it really make in the long run if it takes you an extra month or so to ease into maintenance? After all, you dieted to reach your goal and maintenance will help you stay at your goal weight—forever! ❤

Get Thee Behind Me

Diet devils on the loose! The more progress you make toward being thin, the more diet devils you will attract. Diet devils are well-meaning friends and acquaintances who tell you constantly how great you already look or how skinny you are getting. Although it is very flattering, don't let it tempt you to stray from your weight-loss program. Remember your own goals and repeat after me, **"nothing tastes as good as being thin feels."** ♥

Fast **TRACK**

If it is fast weight loss it probably won't last.
Quick-fix diets, such as losing ten pounds over a weekend, dropping a dress size in only one week, etc. may offer the temptation of a speedy cure, but initially, you are only losing water, not fat.
STUDIES SHOW THAT WITH THESE TYPES OF DIETS, THE WEIGHT LOST IS BACK ON IN NO TIME.♥

DANGER

ADVANTAGE

If a certain time of the day is deadly for your diet,

WHY not SCHEDULE that time

FOR exercise? By having a plan, you gain

control, plus at the end of the exercise session, you

will feel empowered and energized. ♥

162

Not a Hobby

LOSING WEIGHT SHOULD NOT BE A HOBBY.

If you have been down the weight-loss road before, you know that it takes persistence and determination, while a hobby is what you do to relax or keep entertained. *Aren't there better hobbies than dieting?* Determine how this time losing weight will be different for you. ❤

TIME DELAYS

Instead of streamlining activities, such as one trip from the car to the kitchen with all of the groceries, or assembling all that is needed for a project before beginning, **GET IN THE HABIT OF MULTIPLE TRIPS.** Gathering needed items in small loads will burn more calories. Also, opt for good old-fashioned labor to do chores instead of using all of those labor-saving devices. Keep that body moving! ❤

Score **TWO POINTS**

Make it a habit to **scrape all the leftovers on the plate into the trash.** The last bite of your child's hotdog or ketchup-seasoned fries is just not worth it. Save those calories for something that you will really enjoy! ♥

PUSH

Truer Words
WERE NEVER SPOKEN

"If you keep doing what you've done, you will keep getting what you've got."

Staying the same is not an option. Take control of all elements of your weight loss: **1)** *food plan,* **2)** *exercise program,* **3)** *thought patterns,* **4)** *self-improvement activities.* Now you are really thinking. ❤

166

WEAK Ends

Weekends may be hazardous to your waistline. A recent study revealed that on average we eat significantly more at the weekend, compared with other days of the week—enough additional calories are added to gain five pounds a year! To prevent weekend weight gain, try limiting alcohol to mealtimes only. **BE AWARE** of what you are putting in your mouth. Also try stepping-up physical activities on the weekends to make the most of the extra time you have. ♥

It's the Truth

If you do the work, the weight loss will come, _you can count on it._ Knowing that you have done all you can do, and practiced what you preach, you will find that the weight-loss universe will reward you. _You'll meet your goals, gain a body you love, and have a future that is unlimited._ ♥

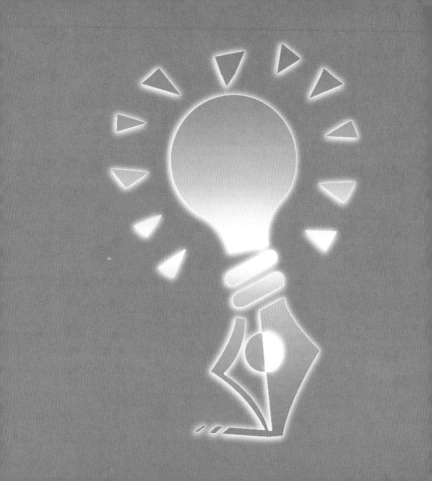

"Life itself is the proper binge."
Julia Child

Food for Thought

This chapter provides true brain food for your weight-loss program. **The tips and techniques included will help make you a wiser and smarter weight-loss planner.** Adding just a bit of this and perhaps a dash of that will make your meal planning easier, plus, increase the health quotient. ❤

171

Sweet Thing

Sweet potatoes are a great source of vitamin A. Vitamin A is a powerful antioxidant and helps to promote BEAUTIFUL SKIN. It

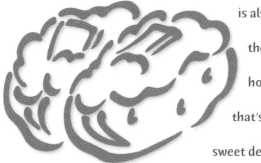

is also essential for the production of hormones. Now that's what I call a sweet deal! ❤

Salute!

Red wine contains heart-healthy resveratrol, a compound that protects against cardiovascular disease and cancer. Pinot Noir contains twice as much of this important ingredient as other red wines. Why not toast yourself with a glass of good-for-you red wine? ♥

SOAK it Up

Tomatoes contain lycopene, a wonderful skin nutrient. To help your body to absorb the lycopene, put a dash of fat, such as olive oil, on the tomatoes. You might also enjoy tomato wedges with a slice or two of low-fat cheese. The  fact is that fat helps to bind the vitamins from the tomato and allows for better absorption into the body's system. ❤

HANDLE *With Care*

The look of your skin can be affected by dieting. To keep the skin radiant while on a weight-loss program, *be sure to add evening primrose oil and vitamin E to your daily supplements.* For even better absorption, take the combination just before lights out. Between the hours of 1 A.M. and 4 A.M., the skin is most receptive to moisture and the supplements can be absorbed more effectively. ❤

AS SIMPLE AS a-b-c

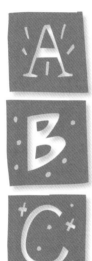

VITAMINS A, B, AND C

are the most important vitamins to help keep hair silky and lustrous, and nails strong and flexible. Make sure that your multi-vitamin contains extra amounts of these important nutrients. Better yet, simply add a vitamin combo specifically made for the nails, hair, and skin. ❤

TOP THIS!

TOP A CUP OF YOGURT WITH A TABLESPOON OR TWO OF A HIGH-FIBER CEREAL, FLAX SEED, OR WHEAT GERM. You will be adding antioxidants, vitamins B and E, and iron for healthy blood cells. Plus, the added fiber is always welcome. ♥

FRUIT Loose

Grab a few raisins and add to your cereal or salad, or have a few orange slices. ***You could even pop some peach or banana slices into your shake,*** or top your fat-free pudding with a berry or two. You will be adding a healthy dose of phytochemicals and polyphenols, plus extra vitamins to boot. ❤

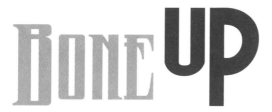

BONE UP

To get even more goodness from your skim milk serving, **TRY ADDING A QUARTER CUP OF NON-FAT DRY MILK AND STIR.** Your calcium intake will be doubled and your milk will have a creamier and richer taste. ❤

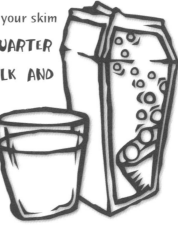

BEAN ME UP

Add beans to soups, stews, or salads. **Beans contain protein and are rich in B vitamins and zinc.** These are all things the body needs to rebuild itself and preserve energy. Plus, beans have no fat content and are an excellent source of fiber. ❤

IT'S a TOSS UP

Add extra veggies to soups, stews, casseroles, and salads as often as possible. THE BENEFITS ARE ENDLESS: vitamins galore, beta-carotene, and phytochemicals. As an added bonus, they taste good too! ❤

Check Your OIL

All oils are high in fat and calories, **BUT OLIVE AND FLAX SEED OILS ARE BETTER FOR YOU BECAUSE THEY PROVIDE OMEGA-3 FATTY ACIDS AND MONOUNSATURATED FATS.** Plus, both contain vitamin E to help protect the skin tissue and cells. ❤

spread *Swap*

Instead of butter or cream cheese, **spread a tablespoon of peanut butter on your bread.** Rich in monounsaturated fat, peanut butter helps to lower cholesterol. Plus, the three to five grams of protein in a tablespoon-sized serving will make you feel full until your next meal. ❤

Fiber-Size IT

Why not increase your fiber intake by trying to eat more **WHOLE-WHEAT** pasta, breads, and cereals. Simply by ditching the cornflakes in the morning and opting for a more fiber-rich cereal, you can add four times the fiber! Think of other ways to increase your fiber throughout the day. ❤

Can It

A three and one-half-ounce serving of canned salmon contains **1,000** milligrams of omega-3 fatty acids, which are excellent cell boosters. As an extra bonus, you will also get **20 percent** of your daily calcium requirement because the salmon contains edible bones. ♥

ALL IN the Wrist

When steeping a tea bag in hot water, you can release more antioxidant compounds into the water by dunking the tea bag up and down. Swirl the bag around in the cup for one to two minutes to release even more goodness. ♥

Pop a TOP

No time to wash, chop, or grate veggies?

POP A TOP OF LOW SODIUM VEGETABLE JUICE FOR A SERVING OF VEGETABLES ON THE GO. Drink and enjoy. ♥

Seeing RED

RED BELL PEPPERS HAVE **ten** TIMES THE AMOUNT OF VITAMIN A AND MORE THAN DOUBLE THE VITAMIN C OF THEIR GREEN COUSINS. Always choose red peppers—those added nutrients are worth it. ❤

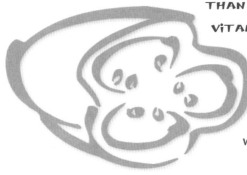

Seize the C

Vitamin C is important in aiding the formation of collagen, which helps to keep your skin firm and sag-free. Choose *vitamin C-rich foods* such as berries, citrus fruits, and dark green vegetables to keep your skin looking its best. ❤

TOFU *for You*

Lower your meat and fat consumption by adding tofu or soybeans to your meals. Soy is a wonderful source of soluble fiber, protein, iron, B vitamins, potassium, zinc, and other essential minerals. Stir-fry some with your favorite veggies or put over brown rice—**tofu terrific!** ♥

190

Say "Okay" to oats

Oatmeal has one of the highest concentrations of protein, calcium, iron, magnesium, zinc, copper, manganese, thiamin, and vitamin E, of any other unfortified whole grain. *Add some oats to your diet by eating a bowl of oatmeal at breakfast or perhaps enjoy your favorite sandwich with oat bran bread.* ♥

OVER the TOP

Instead of using light syrup on your pancakes and waffles, **top with sliced peaches, strawberries, or blueberries.** Another great way to add a little extra boost is to use orange juice in place of the liquid when mixing the pancake or waffle batter. Want even more nutrients? Sprinkle some oatmeal or bran into the batter mixture before cooking. ❤

Blues clues

BLUEBERRIES ARE LOADED WITH ANTIOXIDANTS and studies show that eating half a cup of blueberries a few times a week, *can improve your short-term memory and fight the signs of aging.* ♥

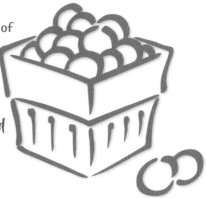

Try Chai

Instead of the usual coffee concoction, try chai. Made from black tea, spices, and steamed milk (ask for skim), this drink provides bone-strengthening calcium and the disease-fighting properties of tea. It also contains small amounts of ginger and cinnamon, two spices that help to soothe the stomach and speed up recovery from cold symptoms. ❤

Preserve *the Produce*

Did you know that cutting produce into small sections exposes the inner surface to air, allowing veggies to oxidize more rapidly and letting valuable vitamins leach out? *So keep the chopping on the coarse side,* and keep those all-important vitamins in. ❤

DRINK ÜP!

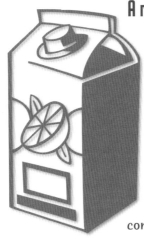

A ready-to-drink carton of orange juice loses up to 45 milligrams of vitamin C per cup, within four weeks of opening the carton. To get all of the healthy benefits of orange juice, be sure to purchase three to four weeks prior to the expiration date on the carton and consume within one week of opening. ❤

Fishing for Compliments

Seafood is loaded with protein, essential fatty acids (EPAs), and omega-3 oils. It is low in fat and is one of the healthiest foods available. Seafood has been shown to decrease the risk of coronary artery disease and to lower cholesterol. Two servings of a relatively fatty fish like tuna, salmon, or mackerel every week can help to lower the risk of developing heart disease. ♥

Dairy Delicious

Calcium, most prevalent in dairy products, has been shown to reduce the chances of being overweight by 75 percent when at least 1,200 milligrams is consumed daily. Compare this with the average daily consumption of only 200 milligrams. Make a date to add dairy to your daily regimen. ♥

Scavenger HUNT

Each week or so, explore the vegetable aisles at your grocery store. Search for little known or untried veggie varieties. Try something new, like bok choy, collards, or maybe even winter squash. Hunt for new fruits while you are at it. Your taste buds will thank you for the experience! ❤

Eat Low and Glow

LOW-GLYCEMIC FOODS, SUCH AS WHOLE GRAINS, LEGUMES, AND SWEET POTATOES, TEND TO BE HIGHER IN FIBER AND COMPLEX CARBOHYDRATES; while high-glycemic foods such as white rice, white breads, and pastas hardly have any fiber. Don't waste your time, or your calories. ❤

No More KiD STuff

Puffed rice, puffed wheat, or corn flakes, while low in the calorie department, lack the fiber you need to start the day on the right foot. **Read the labels and choose cereals with at least three grams of fiber for a better boost to your morning.** ❤

GO NUTS!

Find ways to add nuts to your diet every day. **Nuts are a great source of monounsaturated fats.** Add some almonds, walnuts, or pine nuts to salads, rice, pasta dishes, and vegetable entrées. Studies show that eating five ounces of nuts a week, will make you 45 percent less likely to develop heart disease due to cholesterol. ❤

Only Seeing PURPLE

When you see dark green broccoli, or broccoli with a purplish-color—pick it first! **The purple color is an indication that it is loaded with life-affirming beta-carotene.** Throw out old broccoli that has turned yellow—no nutrients and no good for you! ❤

POPEYE WAS RIGHT

SPINACH IS PACKED WITH HIGH LEVELS OF ANTI-OXIDANTS THAT HELP TO KEEP YOUR MIND SHARP. How about adding some fresh spinach to an omelet, or to a pasta dish, as a slimming, but healthy treat? ❤

"A meal however simple, is a moment of intersection.
It is at once the most basic, the most fundamental, of our life's activities,
maintaining the life of our bodies; shared with others it can be
an occasion of joy and communion, uniting people deeply."
Elise Boulding

Celebrate

Holidays, special occasions, and even life itself are cause for celebration. Enjoy the good times, but don't get carried away and overindulge. With a little pre-party planning, you are sure to be the belle of the ball, without sacrificing your weight-loss goals. ❤

207

IN CONTROL

DURING THE HOLIDAYS do not plan to increase your workouts, **JUST PLAN ON MAINTAINING THEM.** With all the added activities of the holiday season, sticking to your routine will help to keep you in control. ❤

Welcome the SANDMAN

Get plenty of sleep.

During times of celebration, usually the first thing to go is your sleeping schedule. Sleep is the very thing that will help you maintain emotional tolerance—especially when controlling your diet. ♥

UP AND AT 'EM

Start your day on a positive note by exercising first thing in the morning. Don't let the craziness of the holidays interrupt your fitness routine. ❤

IT IS BETTER TO GIVE

If you are hosting a party make sure you have plenty

of takeout cartons—you may even be able to find

some to match your theme. **WHEN**
GUESTS LEAVE, INSIST
THEY TAKE SOME
GOODIES HOME.

Cleaning up will be a breeze

and tons of fat and calories are

out of sight, mind, and house. ❤

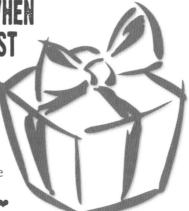

BALANCING 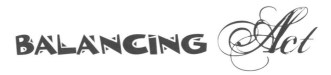Act

At a gathering, try holding your drink with your dominant hand. You are less likely to try and balance a big plate of food with your less dominant hand. ♥

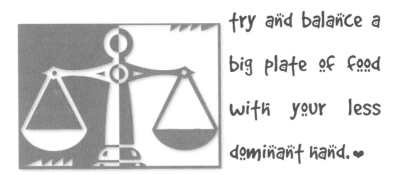

212

LOOK, NO HANDS

SKIP FINGER FOODS. High fat hors d'oeuvres
like cheese puffs, baby quiches,
mozzarella sticks, and the like
are just too tempting.
Exceptions to the rule are
fresh veggies, fruit
slices, and shrimp. ❤

CHOOSE and *Lose*

Survey the entire buffet before deciding what to eat.

If you don't know what's up ahead, you will pick up what's in front of you and before you know it your plate will be full. You can't return items to the buffet and you will probably feel obligated to eat everything on your plate. A little bit of forward planning will help you to save the calories for those things you *really* want. ❤

Savor *the Season*

Choose to pass up the regular everyday snacks

that are at every gathering and

occasion. Opt

instead to *treat*

yourself   to

foods that are

traditional to the

special season. ❤

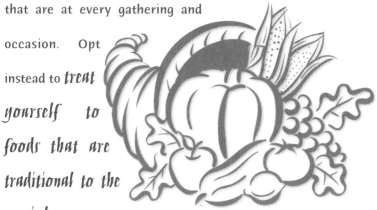

Last CALL

DECIDE TO BE LAST IN LINE FOR THE BUFFET.

You will find all of the really popular fattening items have vanished, leaving only the healthy foods for you. ❤

216

POT Luck

When asked to bring a dish to a party, choose a delicious low-fat, low-calorie dish. Make it colorful and inviting. Chances are you will find that your dish is the first eaten as more and more of us are looking for healthy alternatives! ❤

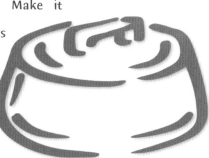

Water versus **ALCOHOL**

FOR EVERY ALCOHOLIC DRINK YOU HAVE,

sip a glass of water, or tonic in between.

This will slow your consumption of

high-calorie alcoholic drinks and keep

you from becoming dehydrated as well. ❤

DISH It Out

If you simply must have a candy dish out for the holidays, choose a candy that you do not like. It's the gesture that counts. As for Halloween candy, don't buy it before the 31st and keep the bag sealed until the Trick-or-Treaters arrive to avoid temptation. ❤

IT'S YOUR Birthday

For birthdays, instead of a birthday cake, pick up some elegant petits fours or even CUPCAKES.

Purchase one for each guest and send any leftovers home with them. Out of sight, out of mind. ❤

Create a Tradition

Instead of an all out holiday meal, why not choose an event or outing as a way of celebrating. **Look in the "what's happening" section of the newspaper and plan a day out.** Who knows, it could become your special holiday tradition. ❤

221

marvelous MASH

Instead of using cream or butter to mash the holiday potatoes, **try blending skim milk, diced garlic, and a dash of Italian seasoning in with them.** The taste will be full and flavorful without the added fat. ❤

COOKIE Caper

When baking holiday cookies, **TRY ADDING EXTRA FIBER, SUCH AS BRAN FLAKES, OAT BRAN, OR EXTRA RAISINS, AND PERHAPS USE APPLE SAUCE INSTEAD OF OIL.** Cookies will be moist, delicious, and good for you too! ♥

Cheers!

champagne contains fewer calories than other alcoholic beverages.

Plus, the natural carbon gas will aid your digestion. A **flute of the bubbly stuff is only about 75 calories.**

Go on, have two glasses. ♥

PARTY ANIMAL

When attending social functions where food and beverages are on offer, **REMIND YOURSELF THAT YOU'RE AT A SOCIAL FUNCTION, NOT AT AN EATING ENGAGEMENT.** Enjoy the company but take control of 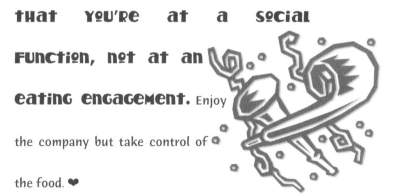 the food. ❤

Social Graces

General principles of a party:

Remember, as soon as you put something in your mouth, someone will **a)** hug you or **b)** ask you a question. Neither one is pretty with a half eaten Swedish meatball still being chomped on in your mouth. Choose easy-to-eat foods and remember— take tiny bites! ❤

Keep it *Light*

Instead of piling on the party platter in one hand, and brandishing a cocktail glass in the other, opt instead for one thing at a time. Start with a vegetable relish, after completing it, move on to a wine spritzer. **Party rule—as you circulate, keep one hand free at all times** in case you need to meet and greet another partier. ❤

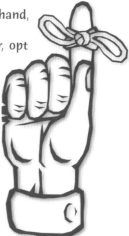

PLATEAU *the* PLATEAU

"Staying the same" in the weight-loss world is called a "plateau." A plateau is nothing to fear. It is just a stopping place to allow the body to catch up to the progress you have made so far. It allows for our "heads" to catch up with our "bodies." Relax and know that if you keep it up, more weight loss will follow. Just give it time and breathe in your success. ❤

TOMORROW, TOMORROW,
I Love You TOMORROW

It's true! Tomorrow is only a day away. If you cannot make the commitment to a week, then tomorrow is the perfect time. If you promise yourself that you will do whatever it takes today for your program, then tomorrow will be easy! ♥

Grand Prix

It takes a mere 500 calories extra a day, from Thanksgiving to New Year's Day, to gain five pounds! Start your brain engine thinking about the extra goodies that are mindlessly added during the holidays. *Rev yourself up* for the weight-loss race. Ask yourself— is this food going to put me in the winner's circle? ❤

LATE COMER

if attending a party where food and alcohol will be the center of attention, *show up late.* Everyone will have nibbled and noshed, toasted and cheered. The new, slimmer you can make a grand entrance. Suddenly you—not the "fare"—will be the center of attention. ❤

Call it **A DAY**

Remember it is a holi-day— not a holi-week or holi-month.

Plan ahead for wise holi-day eating. By all means

enjoy the specialties of the day, but remember

it is only a day, and with good

planning, the scales will still be

balanced come next sunrise. ♥

Let's Do Lunch

LUNCH IS PROBABLY THE BEST TIME TO HAVE A CELEBRATION PARTY. Lunchtime portions are generally smaller than dinner portions, therefore you will eat fewer calories! The best news is that you have the rest of the day to work it off. ❤

DON'T EVEN THINK ABOUT IT

Dessert that is—until you have eaten your main meal. By not thinking about how your meal will end, you may find that your choice changes to something lighter, or maybe nothing at all. ♥

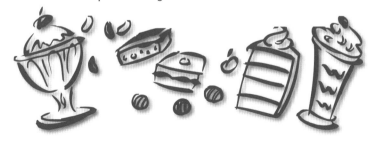

Get REAL

One meal or party will not make or break your weight-loss program, especially if you plan ahead for the indulgence. Maybe during times of celebration, it is more realistic to concentrate on maintaining your success rather than losing more weight. Just a thought. ❤

BE a Sweetheart

If only to yourself. **When Valentine's Day rolls around, gently let it slip that flowers are your absolute favorite things in the whole world.** Or you could even hum "Diamonds Are A Girl's Best Friend" over and over until the hint is taken. If Cupid brings a box of chocolates—take heart, take one piece and put the rest in the freezer, or better yet share with the office as soon as possible! ❤

If You Can—Cater

For your next social gathering, why not call ahead to a health food store, or "guiltless gourmet" takeout place. Whether it is one dish or a full blown meal for your gathering, **BY PLANNING AHEAD** and telling them how you would like the food prepared, you will avoid a "FULL BLOWN" episode of eating off your plan. ♥

237

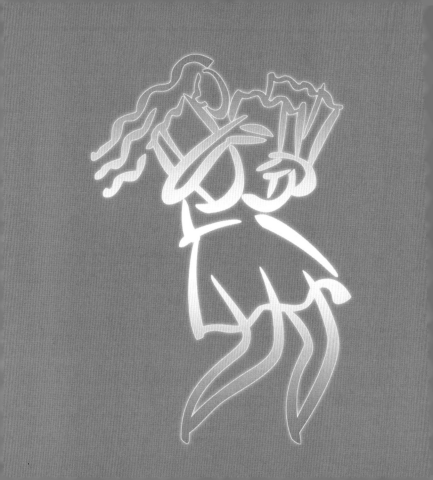

"Never eat more than you can lift."
Miss Piggy

Beauty Bytes

Miss Piggy spoke a lot of sense. Another great quote, **"beauty is as beauty does"** might be considered the theme of this chapter, which shows you clever ways to maintain the flavor of your food, without the extra calories and fat. ♥

239

PILE it ON

Add all the lettuce, tomatoes, cucumber slices, alfalfa sprouts, peppers, onions, and any other fresh vegetables you can think of to top off your sandwich or burger.

You will feel like you have eaten a lot more without adding any extra calories. Plus, the colorful vegetable crunch adds to your satisfaction level. If you pile it on so high that you can't get your mouth around it, just scrape some onto your plate and eat it as a side salad. ❤

Be Prepared

Keeping a couple of treats that you enjoy nearby and accessible could help you to avoid a full-blown snacking binge. Fudge-flavored popsicles in the freezer, a small bag of baked potato chips, or popcorn could be just the answer to satisfy your cravings. ♥

DE-GREASE with Ease

Remove the excess oil from a pizza slice with a paper towel. Press down on the top and repeat to absorb as much of the grease as possible.

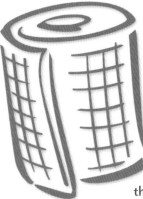

WHEN YOU SEE WHAT THE PAPER TOWEL LOOKS LIKE YOU MAY THINK TWICE ABOUT EATING THE PIZZA.

Or at the very least, you will have the satisfaction of knowing that most of the oil slick has been removed. ♥

242

Chew 'em IF YOU Got 'em

Chewing sugarless gum while preparing meals will help you keep from tasting too much, too soon. The gum-chomping will also help to reduce stress levels. Food that gets stuck in gum is not very appealing—so always chew gum instead of food, while cooking. ♥

Souper!

Add lots of extra veggies—the more the merrier—to canned soups for a more satisfying meal.

If you really want to get creative try adding a little brown rice, some potatoes, and your favorite **"ZIP IT UP"** spices—now it really tastes homemade—in a smidgen of the time. ❤

Quick *Thinking*

Keep **a bag or two of frozen vegetables** in your freezer at all times for when you have run out of fresh veggies—and you need a good meal—quick! Simply pop some of the frozen vegetables into your soup, pasta, omelet, or whatever else suits your cuisine fancy, for an even more healthy meal. ❤

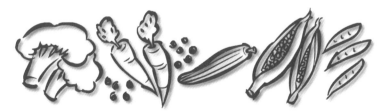

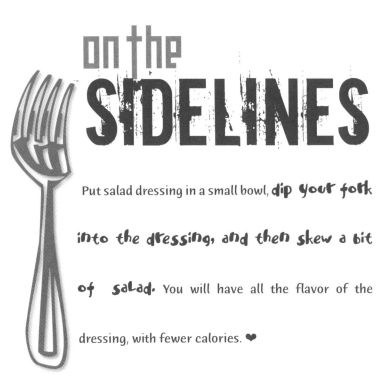

on the
SIDELINES

Put salad dressing in a small bowl, **dip your fork into the dressing, and then skew a bit of salad.** You will have all the flavor of the dressing, with fewer calories. ❤

Less LOOKS LIKE MORE

When baking muffins, try a mini tin that holds **24** instead of **12.** This way you can have two muffins in a serving instead of one. ❤

Join the Club

Cut sandwiches in quarters, à la club sandwich style.

It will look like there is more food on your plate.

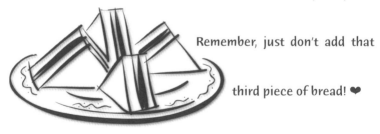

Remember, just don't add that

third piece of bread! ❤

WHAT'S UP DOC?

Baby carrots contain **70 percent** more beta-carotene than their grown-up counterparts. Good, healthy food crunching and more antioxidants to boot. *Now that's a great combination.* ♥

LIVE IT UP SOME

If a chocolate drop or two, or a small cookie make you feel happy—so be it. **ALLOW YOURSELF A SMALL DAILY TREAT—LOOK FORWARD TO IT AND ENJOY IT.** Just remember that too many treats will lead you back to the beginning. ♥

An Appealing TREAT

A banana, **at only 80 calories**, is a naturally sweet and filling way to satisfy your sweet tooth.

As an added bonus, bananas are a great way to add potassium and fiber to your food plan. ❤

Food *Fast*

Instead of grabbing a fast-food meal, opt for a "food-fast" healthy meal. Grocery stores are onto the eating-right trend, carrying foods that are fresh and fast. Pre-packaged salads, prepared meats, salad bars, dinners for two, cooked entrées, and other healthy food selections, can be found throughout most stores. *Think of the fat and calories you will save by choosing a healthy, ready-to-go alternative,* instead of the endless wait in line at the drive-thru—to say nothing of having to yell into a box to order your meal. ❤

Cool IT

When cooking, keep the temperature on the lower side. **By cooking with less heat, you are able to use less oil to prepare a meal.**

High temperatures increase the evaporation factor, tricking you into adding more oil. ♥

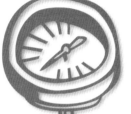

Freshest *of the Fresh*

Make a vow to only eat fresh foods.

"Fresh," as in "prepared recently."

Wilted vegetables, one day past their expiration date and a tiny bit stale are not what healthy eating is all about. You would not serve your guests anything less than the best would you? Treat yourself as a guest in your own home. ❤

Steamed Up

Steaming vegetables saves the vitamin content.

Boiling vegetables depletes the vitamin content substantially. **GET YOURSELF STEAMED UP!** ♥

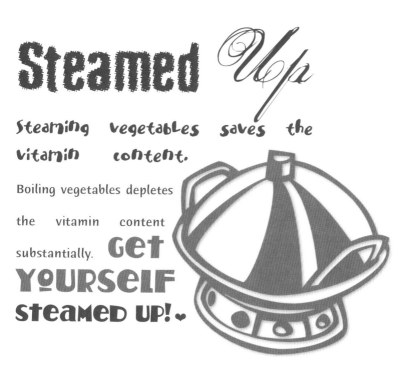

MUSTARD
the Courage

MUSTARD IS AN EXCELLENT WAY TO SPICE UP A SANDWICH INSTEAD OF USING HIGH-IN-FAT MAYONNAISE. Mustard comes in all kinds of varieties—find one that you like and give your meal extra zip. ❤

CELEBRATE CELERY

CRISP, COOL CELERY IS A GREAT LOW-CALORIE SNACK IDEA. It contains fiber and nutrients such as calcium and magnesium. Plus the sound produced by the *crunch as you munch* is very satisfying. ♥

GRATING
IS GRADE A

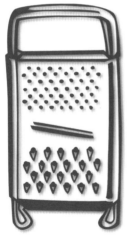

Grating vegetables like carrots, cabbage, celery, cucumber, etc. adds volume to your meals. BY GRATING, YOU CAN CREATE SUPER-SIZE SALADS AND ENJOY SECOND HELPINGS WITH ONLY A FEW EXTRA CALORIES. ♥

Pizzazz
With the Punch

Gourmet jellybeans are a delicious way to get an exotic taste for practically nothing.

If you just have to have the taste of cheesecake, praline, brownies, or even crème brûlée—there is a jellybean somewhere with your name on it. You'll only need a couple to send your taste buds soaring and to satisfy your craving without a speck of guilt. ❤

SEIZE the Seeds

Seeds are loaded with nutrients and fiber.

Sprinkle some sesame or sunflower seeds over salads and vegetables

to instantly add extra goodness and

extra flavor to your meal. ❤

Soy — *Oh Boy!*

INCORPORATING SOY INTO YOUR MEAL PLAN IS AN EXCELLENT WAY TO BOOST YOUR OVERALL HEALTH. Soy is loaded with antioxidants, which help to reduce painful symptoms during your menstrual cycle and even lower blood cholesterol. ❤

Keep the Flavor

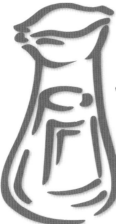

Substitute fatty oils and cream for a little bit of yogurt, vinegar, or a low fat condiment when making your favorite dressing or marinade. You will lower the fat without tossing flavor aside. ♥

BLOAT BANISHER

When you feel puffy and bloated, **try the bloat banisher cocktail.** Put one cup of red cabbage, one apple, one tablespoon of parsley, one carrot, and one celery stick into a blender and thoroughly blend together. Drink a glass of this delicious cocktail up to three times a day to help rid the body of *EXTRA FLUID OR INDULGENCES.* ♥

Stroke OF LUCK

consuming fruits rich in vitamin C,

such as citrus fruits, and eating vegetables that are

high in fiber, such as broccoli, cabbage, Brussels

sprouts, and spinach, is ***excellent for a weight-

loss plan.*** But studies also show that these foods

reduce the likelihood of having a stroke.

Great-tasting foods that are truly good for you. ❤

264

THINK FLAVOR—
Not Fat

Adding black shiitake or portabella mushrooms to an entrée increases the flavor but not the fat. If cheese is called for, choose a small piece of goat's cheese for a flavorful burst. Small amounts of goat's cheese or highly appetizing mushrooms will intensify the flavor without adding any extra fat. ❤

ON THE WHOLE

WHOLE SPICES TASTE BETTER.

Buy whole cumin, mustard, coriander, nutmeg, cinnamon sticks, etc. Put some of the whole spice in a dry skillet and cook for three minutes. Let cool, then grate in a spice mill. The extra burst of flavor will astound you. Store any leftovers in a clean spice jar for future use. ❤

Rotisserie ROULETTE

Self-basting poultry or "**rotisserie style**" PREPARED MEALS ARE USUALLY ABSOLUTELY LOADED WITH EXTRA FAT.

Opt instead for the oven roasted varieties, which have nothing added, for the healthiest possible choice. ♥

SkinFlint

To increase fiber content in meals and snacks, **leave the skin intact** on fruits and vegetables like apples, pears, nectarines, cucumbers, potatoes, eggplants, and carrots, as this is where most of the fiber resides. Just be sure to scrub well before preparing. ❤

Egg-cellent

EGGS ARE, THANK GOODNESS, OFF THE DIETERS ENDANGERED SPECIES LIST—AS WELL THEY SHOULD BE. Eggs are good for you—a great source of protein, vitamin B, and lecithin, a compound that helps with brain functions. **MMMM, OMELETS FOR LUNCH ANYONE?** ♥

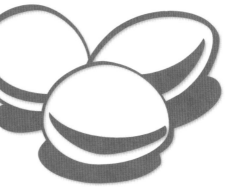

TRYING IT ON For Size

A one-ounce cheese slice is the **size of a computer disk**. One cup of cooked pasta equals the **size of an orange.** A bagel serving is about the **size of a CD**. A slice of pizza should fit into a standard **#10 business envelope,** and a brownie square is about the **size of a business card.** Think about the portion size of your food—remember to keep it all in perspective. ❤

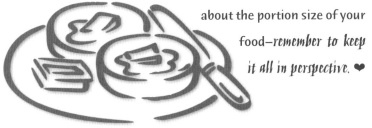

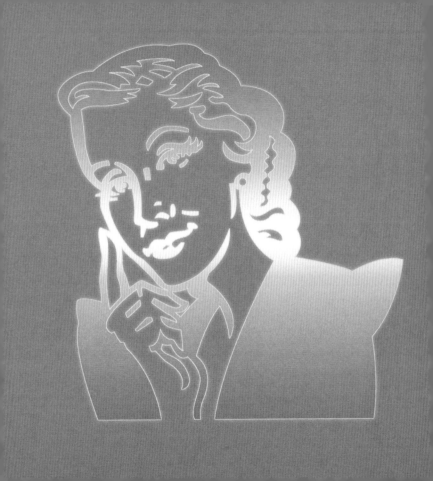

"How we spend our days is, of course, how we spend our lives."
Annie Dillard

Did You Know?

While you may have already heard some of the tips in this chapter, my guess is that **most of what you read here will leave you saying to yourself, "HMMM, I DIDN'T KNOW THAT."** My goal is to have you say **"I CAN DO THAT!"** ❤

IT ALL adds up

If you **subtract 250 calories** from your daily

caloric intake and incorporate exercise that will

burn off 250 more calories

during a workout (such as 45 minutes brisk walking

or 35 minutes of lifting weights) you will lose about

one pound of fat each week. ❤

KEEP it to Two

YOU SHOULD NOT PLAN ON LOSING MORE THAN TWO POUNDS PER WEEK. When you do, you are primarily losing water. You will be dehydrated, not thinner! ❤

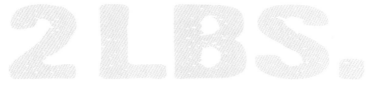

Counts Counter

Keep your calorie count above a minimum of 1,200 calories per day. Dipping below 1,200 will cause side effects such as irritability, nervousness, depression, and even decreased weight-loss results. **Counterproductive to say the least!** ♥

GiveMe **FIVE**

EATING FIVE TIMES DAILY AS OPPOSED TO THE TRADITIONAL THREE SQUARES A DAY, IS HEALTHIER FOR YOU.

Having your food intake spread evenly over five meals has a positive effect on blood insulin levels, which helps control appetite and cravings. ❤

get the skinny
ON THE SKINNY

"REDUCED FAT" means the food item

contains **35 PERCENT** or

less fat than the traditional serving. ♥

LIGHTEN UP

"Light" or "lite" means the item contains one-third fewer calories and/or 50 percent less fat than the "regular" kind. ♥

FREE
AT LAST

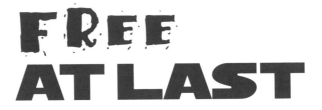

"Fat *free"* means that the item has under one-half a gram of fat per serving. ♥

LOW DOWN

Low **FAT** is when a food contains

three grams of fat or less

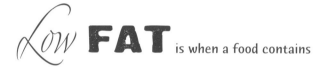

per serving. ❤

count 'em

"*Low* calorie"

means the item contains LESS

THAN 40 CALORIES

PER SERVING. ♥

LEAN and MEAN

"*Lean*" is under ten grams of fat and only four and one-half grams or less of saturated fat.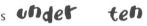

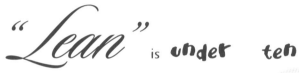

283

OFF TO A GOOD START

Eating a nutritious breakfast everyday will allow you to metabolize food better for the rest of the day. This in turn will help with weight loss since the food is used as fuel and not stored as fat. ❤

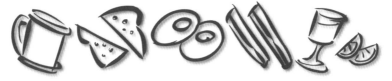

Lose the Diet

People who have been successful in both losing the weight and keeping it off have done so by continuing with the plan of action that helped them lose the weight in the first place.

Maintenance

includes watching portions, fat and calories, and maintaining an exercise program. ❤

TIMING **Is Everything**

One study followed the eating trends of people of various weights and monitored when they ate. Researchers discovered that overweight people tended to eat more of their meals late in the day compared to people of average weight. Make it a habit to eat early and resist late night munching. ♥

Nuke the Myth

Contrary to popular belief, **microwave cooking doesn't zap vitamins.** In fact, less vitamin value loss occurs when cooking food in a microwave. It is because the microwave current passes through the food without heat. ❤

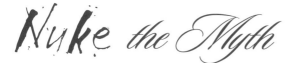

Sightseeing

The average refrigerator is opened

23 times a day, just so we can

stare inside. Most of the time the

door is opened out of boredom,

not because of hunger. **Keep**
it closed and get
a hobby! ♥

ICE COLD

You burn up to 100 extra calories by drinking iced water as opposed to water at room temperature.

Your metabolism will be revved up in order to warm the water so that the body is able to use it. **NOW THAT'S REALLY COOL!** ♥

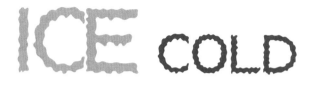

Chill OUT

Sleeping in a slightly cooler room than you are used to can aid in burning extra calories. To offset the cooler temperature, the body compensates by burning more calories to keep warm. ♥

Souped UP

By starting a meal with a cup of soup, hunger pangs are eased. Studies show that beginning a meal with **soup helps save up to 300 extra calories** because as the initial hunger is satisfied the tendency to overeat is as well. ❤

Wake Up *and* SMELL THE COFFEE

A cup of good homebrewed coffee has less than five calories, while a café mocha from your favorite coffee bar has at least 150! WOW! Stay away from those high-calorie splurges—save a little money *and* your figure. ❤

Sweet Tooth

Have an unending craving for something sweet?

Curb it with a piece of hard candy.

At under **30** calories, the candy slowly melts in

your mouth and you can enjoy it for **15** minutes—

that's about **two** calories a minute. By the time

it has melted, the cravings will have too. ❤

SLEEPING BEAUTY

Sleep, and plenty of it, is a necessary tool for dieting success. When you don't get enough sleep, your tired body compensates by storing or craving fat. This means that you will probably lose the willpower battle and be tempted by fatty foods. *To lose more— sleep more!* ♥

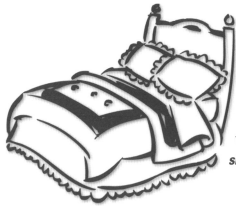

CALORIES *Do Count*

Whether your plan is points, fat grams, pre-packaged, food combining, or any other program—*calorie content will figure into the dieting equation somehow.*

A calorie is simply a measure of energy, energy that the body needs to maintain a constant temperature and perform all of its basic functions. Too many calories in a day? Extras will be stored as fat. Add activities—use more calories. **It is as simple as that.** ♥

WHO COUNTS THOSE THINGS?

A person at their ideal weight has about 30 billion fat cells throughout their body. A person who is 100 pounds or more overweight could have as many as 250 billion fat cells hanging around, and *like a game show prize,* "the cells are yours to keep." *Losing weight reduces the actual fat cell size, but they never go away.* Even worse, if you gain weight you will add even more fat cells to help store the extra fat. **Talk about unfair!** ❤

Figure IT OUT

For each pound you lose, you use **3,500** calories. If you decrease your eating by **70** calories a day, it will take you **50** days to lose one pound. Increase your exercise to burn **175** calories a day, the one pound is gone in **20** days. An ideal weight loss is about **one** to **two** pounds a week. Figure out what you will need to do to get there and make a plan to do it. ❤

NO SWEAT

EVEN IF YOU ARE NOT SWEATING WHILE YOU ARE EXERCISING,

you still need to sip on water during your workout session. When exerting yourself, your muscles release lactic acid, a toxin that can cause muscle fatigue. Drinking water helps to flush the acid from the body. ❤

BATTER UP!

A cup of soup or stew, breakfast cereal, or beans should be about the size of a base-ball. In order to win the weight-loss game, **it is important to step up to the plate** with realistic portion sizes. ♥

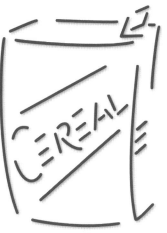

PROOF *of the* PROOF

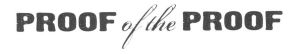

the higher the proof of the liquor, **THE HIGHER THE CALORIES.** If you are having a hard time choosing what to drink, check the label and choose the lower proof. ♥

300

Keep it Personal

Studies show that the most successful dieters don't use expensive programs, **take** pills, **or eat special foods.** The successful majority chooses programs that are easy to follow and tailored to their lifestyle.

Put Some PEP IN YOUR STEP

Regular physical activity makes arteries more elastic, which in turn can make them less prone to hardening. Studies suggest that this beneficial effect could last into a person's 90s!

Remember, move it or lose it! ♥

Focus on Food Groups

two-thirds of the calories in cheese and one-half of the calories in beef come from saturated fat. In contrast, one-third of the calories in pork and one-fourth of the calories in poultry or fish come from saturated fat. Definitely something to focus on when choosing a meal. ❤

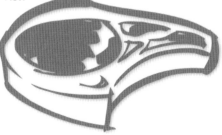

Whining About Wine

A 750 MILLILITER BOTTLE OF WINE HAS 780 CALORIES!

That's only four glasses of vino if using a six-ounce glass. When socializing, it is easy to sip your way through several glasses. *Choose calories wisely.* ♥

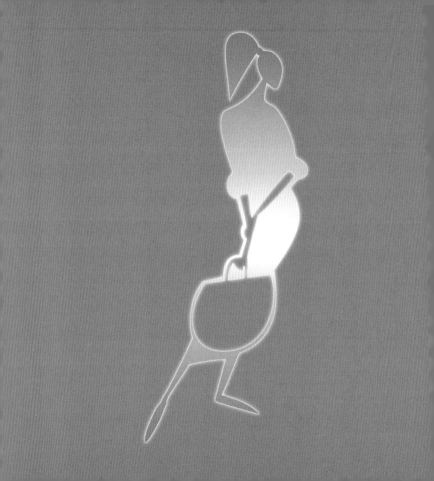

"I don't want to change my life, just my butt."
Julia Roberts

Fooling the Eye

Dressing slimmer is simply smoke and mirrors. **this chapter is filled with tips to help accentuate your assets while playing down the areas that are still under construction.** You will find helpful hints to add value to your figure without adding an ounce of excess baggage! ❤

Basic **BLACK**

They don't call it the "little black dress" for nothing.

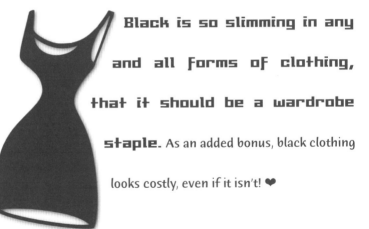

Black is so slimming in any and all forms of clothing, that it should be a wardrobe staple. As an added bonus, black clothing looks costly, even if it isn't! ❤

KEEP it *Light*

Bulky or heavy clothing adds pounds to the figure.

And the sound that corduroy and leather makes as thighs rub together— well, let's just say, it's not pretty. Fabrics that flow and gently skim the body make one appear lighter and thinner. Steer clear of thick and chunky fabrics.

Lighten up. ❤

SHORT BOOTS *and* SKIRTS DO NOT MIX

Your legs will appear WIDER

and shorter. If a monochromatic color

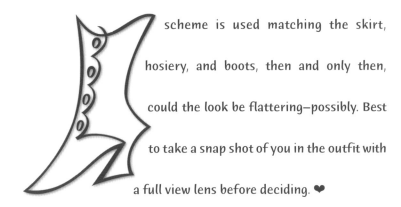

scheme is used matching the skirt,

hosiery, and boots, then and only then,

could the look be flattering—possibly. Best

to take a snap shot of you in the outfit with

a full view lens before deciding. ❤

Best Foot FORWARD

SHOES WITH A BIT OF A HEEL **(TWO TO THREE INCHES)** ELONGATE THE LEGS AND BODY. Also, shoes that have a vamp closer to the toes, such as a v-shaped or rounded curve toward the toes, tend to slim the look of the feet and legs. ❤

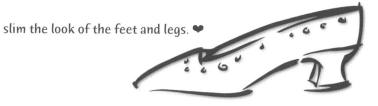

JUST SAY "No"

Shoes with straps or ribbons tied at the ankle are only flattering to someone who is a size six, in clothes and shoes—TRUST ME. ♥

Classic Case

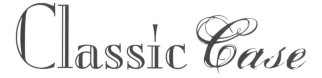

Timeless, tailored garments are much more slimming

than keeping up with the latest fashion

trend. *Keep current,*

but classic, for the

SLIMMEST

silhouette around. ❤

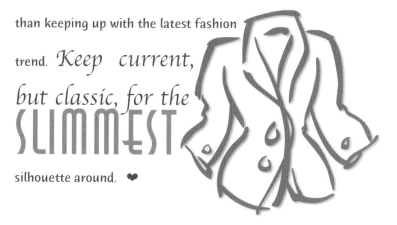

ALL FOR ME

ONE-COLOR OR MONOCHROMATIC DRESSING,

gives your frame an instantly taller and thinner

look. Choose black, navy, gray, or another dark,

receding color to dress in from head to toe. ♥

Top it Off

To keep attention on your face and off your body, **WEAR COLORFUL ACCESSORIES SUCH AS UNIQUE EARRINGS, STRANDS OF PEARLS CRESTING AT THE COLLARBONE, OR TIE A SASSY SCARF AT THE NECK-LINE.** Try an antique necklace, not only beautiful but a great conversation starter as well. ❤

straight and NARROW

A LONG NECKLACE AROUND THE NECK OR LONGER SCARF FLOWING TO THE WAISTLINE CREATES A THINNER LOOK TO THE TORSO. Be careful to keep other accessories to a minimum in order not to appear extra bulky. ❤

Bang It

Wispy bangs are very flattering and slimming to the face.

Be sure to keep them on the

light side. Heavy full bangs will

make the face look shorter

and rounder. ❤

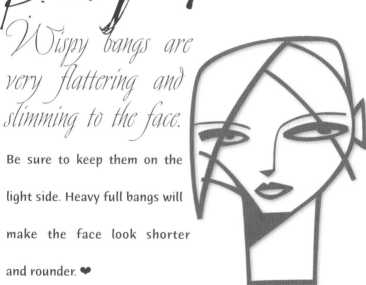

SKIRT *the Issue*

For the most slimming skirt hem length, choose above mid-calf.

Avoid the mid-point of the calf, which is generally

the widest part, as it will make your legs look

heavier. Instead opt for above the knee, knee

length, or go long with the hem cresting on the

lower part of the calf. ❤

EMPTY YOUR POCKETS

Carrying items in pockets adds visual weight to your hips and thighs. INSTEAD, WHY NOT PUT EVERYTHING IN A FLATTERING AND STYLISH HANDBAG? ❤

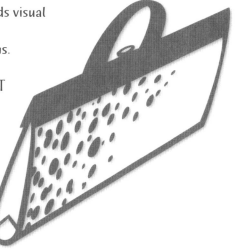

Push UPS

Pushing or rolling up your sleeves is slimming to the torso.

The area between the elbow and waist creates a visual impact of thinness. Add a beautiful bracelet to draw the eye to where you want it to go. ❤

Look Expensive

Invest a little more in your clothes. Pricier items feel more luxurious, drape better, and are apt to be more true to size than cheaper counterparts. ***Invest in looking great—everyday!*** ❤

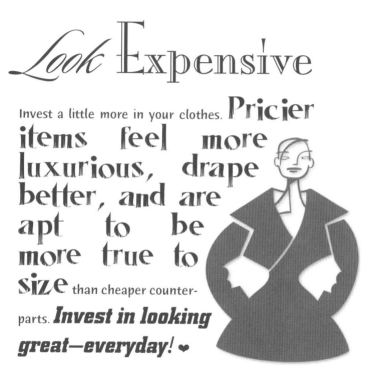

FLAT Out

Pants and skirts without pleats

are much more flattering. Pleats add

unwanted inches to the middle. How many of us

need that? ❤

shape OF THINGS TO COME

If you want to smooth out extra lumps and bumps to create a slimmer silhouette, try a body shaper. Unlike the old-fashioned constricting girdle, *a body shaper simply creates a smoother look to the waist, hips, thighs, and bum, by holding everything firm!* Shapers come in several lengths, some end at the thigh, some at the knee, and some go all the way to Capri length—which is perfect for close-fitting pants. ♥

L**ONG** and **SHORT OF IT**

Pair longer blouses, or separates with short skirts.

Long skirts look more slimming with shorter

blouses or jackets. **long with short**

will keep the silhouette from

looking like it is cut in half. ♥

WARM SHOULDER

Shoulder pads are great for balancing out body proportions.

They come in all shapes and sizes, and unlike the exaggerated pads of the '80s and '90s, current styles add just the right touch of angling to the body. ♥

THE RIGHT *Foundation*

Undergarments should fit correctly for the most slimming look under clothes. Bra straps or waistbands that are too tight will leave red marks after removing. Treat yourself to a proper fitting. You will be amazed at how good you look and more importantly how good you feel. ❤

326

BAG IT

Handbags should complement the figure. A tiny little bag carried by a big woman is not in proportion. Instead choose a good-sized handbag. Keep the straps higher than the hipline for the smallest overall silhouette appearance. A bag resting on the hips just adds extra "baggage" to this all too noticeable area. ❤

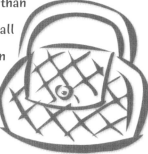

Match It

Hosiery color that matches shoe color creates a longer, leggier look. FOR EVEN MORE OF A *slimming look,* TRY TO MATCH THE HOSIERY AND SHOES TO THE SKIRT OR DRESS HEM-COLOR. This is one of the most flattering looks around. ❤

NIP *It*

Create a gentle inward curve at the waistline. This could be via a tucked-in blouse, a sweater that has a binding type of hem ending at the waistline, or a belt cinching the waistline.

These tips will produce an hourglass look to the figure and show off your curves! ❤

Button **U** **P**

Garments with buttons aligned vertically on the

seam create a nice line that gives the illusion of

a taller, and leaner you. It doesn't matter if you

button up the garment or leave it open—

having the buttons in a straight line will slim the figure. ♥

HIGHLIGHTS

Highlights in the hair and especially those framing the face area illuminate the skin and draw the eye away from the body. Also, streaky highlights create a long thin line to the hair that is carried all the way down toward the body. ❤

331

Slight of Hand

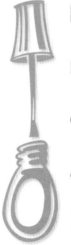

Light-color nail polish or a French manicure adds length to shorter chubby hands. Darker colors have a tendency to emphasize the roundness. For a lean look—go light. ♥

D░ the 'Do

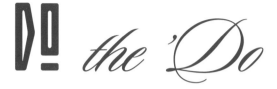

Try a new hair stylist—one who doesn't know you. **Ask them to try a completely new hairstyle.** Something that will flatter the new or almost new you. Enjoy the compliments you'll get and notice that the emphasis is on your hair and not on the areas still under reconstruction. ❤

Tailor Made

Changing dress sizes occurs with every 12 to 18 pounds lost. *Invest in a good tailor who can keep your clothes flattering* and advise you when it's time to donate a box or two of outfits to a good cause. ♥

334

Nifty KNITS

With cotton, silk, or wool knits, you have some sizing leeway as these materials readily adapt to different body sizes.

This will allow you to wear some knits longer than their fabric counterparts. This is really helpful as you go through the in-between sizes stage. ❤

SEEING *Double*

Double chins are more pronounced when hair is pulled back, away from chin and neck. Opt for a hairstyle in which hair is swept toward the chin line and keep it soft and layered, since straight angle cuts, such as the bob style, will draw attention to this problem area. ❤

TEST SPIN

TO GET THE BEST FIT AND MOST FLATTERING STYLE— ALL GARMENTS MUST BE TRIED ON. Catalogs are nice to flip through to get an idea of what you are looking for but clothes need to be seen from all mirror angles. If you simply must have the catalog item, make sure the catalog offers a friendly return policy. ❤

THE GREAT GAP

BLOUSES AND JACKETS MUST NOT BE SO SMALL AS TO HAVE THE BUTTONS OR SNAPS PULL OPEN. Be sure to "road test" the garment by sitting down, and by reaching up to the left and right. In fact, see what you look like in all positions by testing them out in front of the dressing room mirror. ❤

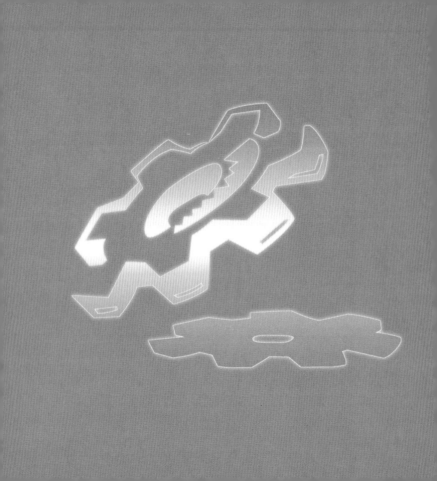

> *"It is better to wear out than to rust out."*
> **Frances E. Willard**

Get Moving

Did you know that less maintenance is required on machinery that is used on a regular basis? Motion keeps the parts from rusting because as the machine moves, each joint and socket is lubricated. **We humans are like the machines that we design and build.** Simple, steady movement will keep our parts rust-free and fuel our souls. An added bonus—slimmer and trimmer outer "machines." ❤

BEGIN in the Beginning

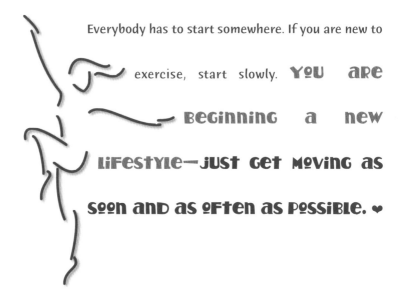

Everybody has to start somewhere. If you are new to

exercise, start slowly. **YOU ARE**

BEGINNING a new

LIFESTYLE—JUST GET MOVING AS

SOON AND AS OFTEN AS POSSIBLE. ❤

Without End

Don't think of exercise as the means to an end. Good, healthy exercise should never stop. **Keep exercising as you grow older to keep you feeling young.** ♥

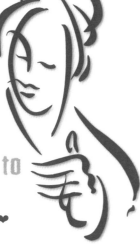

IT ONLY GETS *Better*

Just beginning to exercise? Remember that all of the folks you see on TV and in magazines with great bodies had to start somewhere and you can too! Just put one foot in front of the other and get moving. **The strength and vitality will come.** Trust me, things can only get better. ❤

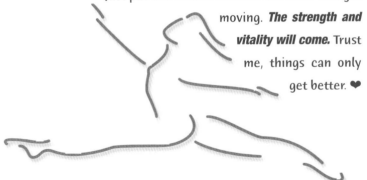

In CONTROL

Take time to learn your exercise routine.

Feel which muscles you're using and how good it feels to move. Contract and release.

Feel the power. Be in control! ♥

Form Fitting

Make sure you have the proper "form." **Form is having the body properly aligned for the exercise to be done.** This must be done for every exercise. If you are unsure about how the body should look while this movement is done, watch a video, study a photograph, or ask your trainer. Do not take shortcuts. This will ensure that you are working the muscles properly for the maximum results. ❤

346

WEIGH *the Odds*

Plan on changing the weight levels with every workout, or at least with every other workout.

By switching it up a notch at regular intervals,

you will be maximizing each workout and achieving

the best results. ❤

Forget the Hare—
Remember the Turtle

Sure and steady is the way. *The most common mistake when exercising is to attempt to become super-fit right away after months, or possibly even years of inactivity.*

This overly zealous attempt will only lead to soreness, frustration, injury or throwing in the towel all together and quitting. Set a reasonable time, about 30 minutes of walking or 20 minutes on the treadmill, etc. and increase it when you feel comfortable. ❤

Calf It Up

WHILE IN THE ELEVATOR OR ON THE ESCALATOR WHY NOT DO SOME CALF RAISES?

People are so busy staring at the floor or the ceiling

that they'll never notice you raising and lowering

your heels. Don't forget to breathe correctly. ❤

Keep the Remote—Remote

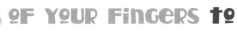

Use Foot Power instead of Your Fingers to Channel Surf.

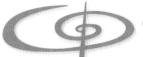

A few trips to the TV and back will burn more calories and prevent you from remaining sedentary. ❤

GET IN THE SWING OF THINGS

Get in the habit of swinging your arms while you walk. You will raise your heart rate, breathe more deeply, and get more energy with each step. Plus, it makes the exercise time fly by. ♥

PUT ON YOUR
Boogie Shoes

Fast dancing for one hour burns over 400 calories. This is almost twice the number of calories burned when walking for the same amount of time.

So get into the groove! ♥

DON'T CRAMP YOUR STYLE

Some women stop exercising during their menstrual

cycle, feeling that working out will only compound

the cramps. Actually just the opposite occurs.

Exercise eases muscle contractions

and helps with the menstrual flow. ❤

HIT *the Spot*

While exercise machines target trouble areas and tighten muscles—only cardiovascular exercise can fight fat. Machines and cardiovascular exercise are the best for maximum results. **A balanced combination of machines and aerobic exercises will maximize your results.** ♥

MOVE the Mood

Studies show that **exercising for as little as 20 minutes can help to raise your mood by 25 percent.**

To feel better both physically and mentally, get

moving. To feel great, keep going! ❤

Backup *Plan*

TO STRENGTHEN BACK MUSCLES and to help rid the area of over-the-top bra bulges, try this exercise. Press your shoulder blades inward, toward your back's middle. Be sure that your posture is erect and correct. **Hold the squeeze for 30 seconds and then release. Repeat ten times.** Make it a habit to do this exercise at least four times a day. It is perfect if you are stuck in traffic, or reading tons of e-mails! ❤

FILM FEST

Before investing in exercise videos, ***check them out at the library or rent a couple at the video store.*** This way you can see if the instructor's style is motivating to you and if you like it enough to persist with it. If the answer to both questions is yes, buy it. ❤

357

Check It Out

Most full service rental companies carry exercise equipment that you can rent for short periods of time, as little as one month. This will give you a chance to see if the treadmill, stationary bike, or whatever piece of equipment you have chosen, is something you will use on a regular basis or if it's destined to become an extra closet rod for clothes. ❤

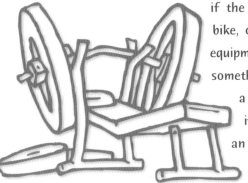

Kick It Up a Notch

Raising the intensity of an exercise by a few notches on the treadmill; pedaling one mile farther on the bike; or walking just a bit faster, will increase your body's metabolic rate by ten percent. Try it and see for yourself. ♥

Waiting to Exhale

When doing strength training, aerobic exercises, or anything else for that matter, you need to breathe. But what is the best way? **To get the most from your effort, breathe in on the up cycle (the beginning) and slowly exhale as your muscles are completing the work.** ❤

Invest In Dress

Invest in proper exercise clothing.

At the top of the list should be proper fitting shoes and for women, always make sure you buy a good workout bra. Instead of grabbing an old bra from your drawer, spend some time and money being fitted correctly. Exercise will be much more comfortable and enjoyable. ❤

Go SLOW

If you want to lose more inches, exercising at a lower intensity works more efficiently. Instead of racing through a routine, take your time to exercise for longer. You will burn the same amount of calories, but studies show that the "slow and steady" group of exercisers doubled the inches lost compared to the "fast and furious." ❤

Walking Papers

Studies show that people who start a simple walking program tend to stick with it. The fall out rate for other exercise programs is double that of walking. **Start walking and make it a habit.** ❤

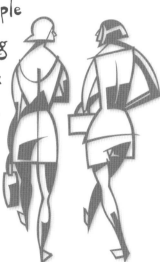

BARGAINS ABOUND

If the cost of exercise equipment is an issue, you can get almost any piece of fitness gear at a second hand store or yard sale. Most of the time the seller has not met their fitness goals—and has given up. That is motivation enough to keep up the exercising—don't you think? ❤

THE LONG and the Short of It

Take the long way. **ANYTIME YOU WALK OR BIKE, TAKE THE SCENIC ROUTE INSTEAD OF THE SHORTCUT.** Whether it is to the break room, the boardroom, or to the mailbox—take the longer route and burn up several more calories as you go. ❤

Don't Be Fooled

Calorie counters on cardio machines can over-estimate the calories burned during exercise by as much as **25 percent.**

The machines are programmed for standard formulas that do not consider variables such as height, fat percentage, or lean muscle mass. It just might take longer than you thought to work off all of last night's indulgence. ❤

Don't HOLD YOUR BREATH

When strength training, it is important not to hold your breath. *Holding your breath could make your blood pressure rise very quickly, causing sudden dizziness or fainting.* Breathe in for two counts while lifting the weight, and exhale for two counts as you are lowering it. Remember to pace yourself and breathe. ❤

Go to the **HEAD OF THE CLASS**

If you have found your exercising niche, be it aerobics, kick boxing, yoga, etc. **why not take an extra credit and become certified in your favorite discipline and perhaps opt to teach a class or two**. That way you will get a great workout by knowing all of the correct moves, plus you will be helping others reach their fitness goals. Grade: **A+.** ♥

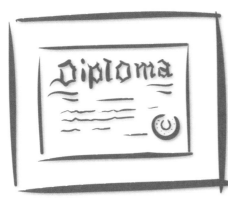

Feel Like a Kid Again

HuLa-hooping is a terrific

workout. Even for just ten

minutes a day, abs will become stronger

and leaner, and hips will get firmer—

all the while you will be smiling. Be a kid again! ❤

Countdown to Curves

When you think, **"this is it, I can't lift another weight or do another sit up,"** remember, it will only take a few more seconds to help create the body you want, so count it down to completion. ♥

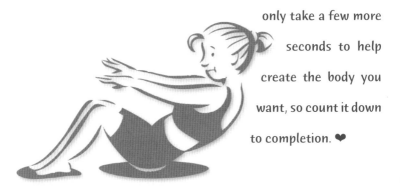

SUIT UP for Success

IF EXERCISING IS ON YOUR CALENDAR FOR TODAY, GET UP AND GET DRESSED FOR YOUR WORKOUT, NO MATTER WHAT OTHER THINGS YOU HAVE TO DO BEFORE YOU EXERCISE. In the event that a phone call runs longer than planned, or surfing the web for ten minutes turns into one hour, you won't wimp out on working out. You will already be suited up for success—now just get moving. ❤

Keep it **HANDY**

If preparing for exercise involves setting up a space,

chances are you will skip it more times than not.

Keep a storage bin accessible containing weights, step, videos, bands, mat, etc.

Bring it out and let

the workout begin. ❤

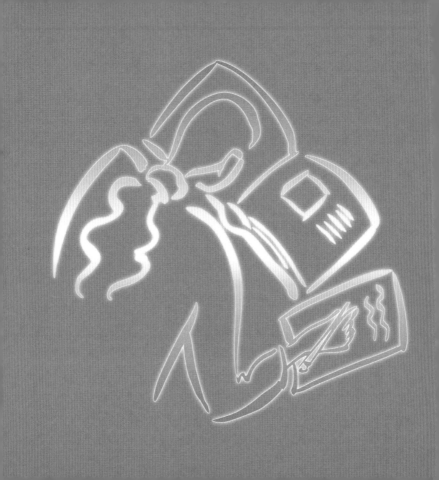

CHAPTER 12

"The ideal life is to do everything a little, and one thing a lot."
Mignon McLaughlin

Keeping Up Appearances

There is no need to stop enjoying your favorite recipes. This chapter shows you how to eat them with weight-loss ease. A smidgen less here, a slight variation there, and you will keep the family traditions intact without the excess fat and calories. ♥

Family TIES

Most likely, an old family recipe passed down from generation to generation will contain unnecessary fat such as butter, oils, or shortening. With today's low-fat alternatives, you can usually safely cut the fat by one-quarter or even one-third and still retain the **"OLD-FASHIONED GOODNESS."** See what new heirloom recipes you can create. ♥

NUTS TO YOU

When nuts are included in a recipe, chop them finely and you will only need about one-half of what the recipe calls for. No one will ever know what's missing. After all, it is the taste you are after, not the extra calories. ❤

DON'T LOSE YOUR COOKIES

TWO REGULAR SIZE CHOCOLATE CHIP COOKIES ONLY HAVE SIX MORE CALORIES THAN THEIR "LOWER FAT" COUSINS. This is because extra sugar is added to the reduced fat cookies in place of the fat. Some savings are just not worth it. Read labels and decide for yourself. After all, you are in the driver's seat. ❤

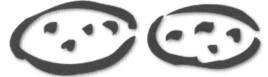

MORE *is Less*

Instead of two and one-quarter cups of pasta at about 450 calories, have one cup of pasta mixed with one cup of steamed vegetables and one cup of steamed, sliced mushrooms. Total calories equals 220. Colorful, filling, and good for you to boot! ❤

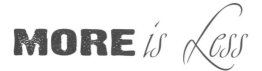

DIVIDE IN HALF =
GET MORE

One cup of granola has about **500** calories.

You could enjoy **ONE AND**

ONE-HALF cups of oatmeal

and even add a small banana or peach for about

250 calories.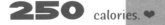

LIGHT WHITES

to reduce your fat intake, opt for doubling the egg whites instead of using the whole eggs that are called for in a recipe. The dish will be light and fluffy without the extra fat and cholesterol. ♥

BOX TOPS

Cut in half the amount of butter or oil called for in boxed side dishes such as rice, macaroni, potatoes, or other starchy foods. Instead, add extra onions, carrots, celery, or other vegetables, and don't forget those spices. The dish will be tasty and satisfying without the extra fat. ❤

SHAKE IT Off

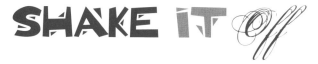

Why choose a fat-laden, sugar-overloaded, milk shake **when all you have to do is blend together your favorite fruits, one cup of skim milk, and one tablespoon of vanilla-flavored whey protein powder.**

Your shake will be creamy, smooth, and wonderfully thick. As you enjoy, think about all of the fat and sugar you are *not* putting in your body. Now that's smooth! ❤

Sauté Savvy

Keep chicken and beef bouillon cubes on hand to make easy, flavorful broths.

Consider these no-fat cubes as

an alternative to fat or

butter to sauté vegetables

and meat dishes. ❤

On the whole

when choosing bread, keep it whole-wheat rather than the nutrition-devoid white variety. Whole-wheat bread at only 65 calories a slice, brings with it magnesium, iron, manganese, zinc, and chromium, which help to build and maintain strong bones. It is also full of the B-vitamin group, which will help you maintain your emotional balance. Plus, it also tastes richer and therefore is more satisfying. ♥

Toss it Up

Instead of greasy croutons, why not crumble a garlic-flavored ricecake on top of your salad?

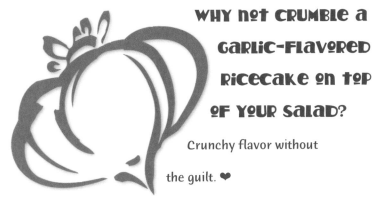

Crunchy flavor without the guilt. ❤

Say "EH?"

Canadian bacon is a delicious alternative to regular fat-laden bacon. Two thick slices of Canadian bacon has only four grams of fat, tons of flavor, and a total of 85 calories—now that's a bacon bargain! ❤

Double the SAVINGS

By choosing pineapple packed in its own juice instead of syrup, you will save at least one-half the calories. As an added bonus, you can sprinkle the juice over any dish to add fat-free zest. ❤

EVAPORATE the fat

Many soup, casserole, and sauce recipes call for cream. **INSTEAD, USE FAT-FREE EVAPORATED MILK.** Rich flavor and zero fat. ♥

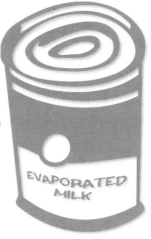

EVAPORATED MILK

Just Add water

If fat-free salad dressings do not appeal to you, simply mix your favorite regular dressing with a drop of water or a touch of vinegar. You'll use less dressing and have the full flavor you love, but with fewer of the unnecessary extra calories. ❤

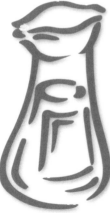

MORE for Less

Instead of a small serving of greasy fast-food french fries, try this idea. Thinly slice a medium baking potato, spray with non-fat cooking oil, and bake at 450 degrees until golden brown and crispy. You've knocked out 50 percent of the calories, and kept 110 percent of the taste. ♥

Say CHEESE

When a recipe calls for cheese, you can reduce the required amount by using intensely flavored cheeses such as parmesan, gorgonzola, and even sharp, white cheddar.

These cheeses pack a powerful flavor so less is needed, yet the dish is still full of creamy richness. ❤

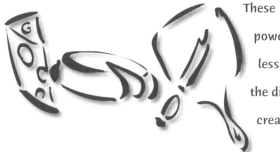

AIN'T NOTHING LIKE
the Real Thing

If only the **"Real Thing"** will satisfy you, then by all means eat it, but choose a smaller serving and really enjoy the experience. **IF ICE CREAM IS YOUR PASSION, INSTEAD OF A REGULAR-SIZE SCOOP, HAVE TWO SCOOPS THE SIZE OF A MELON BALL.**

Pick the flavor of your dreams and put it in a beautiful serving dish. Eat with a demitasse/espresso spoon and savor every bite. ❤

Taking Stock

Toss cooked pasta in a little chicken stock before adding any sauce. The stock adds a smooth texture, and like oil, lubricates the pasta and keeps the strands from sticking together. **Delicious and no fat.** ❤

Sprinkle and **spread**

WHEN MAKING A PIZZA, **TRY GRATING THE CHEESE VERY FINELY. ALSO, EXPERIMENT WITH DIFFERENT TYPES OF CHEESE. DON'T JUST STICK TO MOZZARELLA.** For an extra flavor boost, grate a bit of garlic into the grated cheese. You will find that you need less cheese and that its flavor is more robust. ❤

Sweet Treats Deceit

EXCELLENT LOW-FAT DESSERT CHOICES ARE:

gingersnap cookies or graham crackers dipped in

non-fat whipped topping; a slice of angel food cake

topped with fresh raspberries; or a small fig

bar topped with a small amount of low-fat

peanut butter. LESS THAN 100

CALORIES, BUT 110 PERCENT OF

DELICIOUS, SATISFYING TASTE. ❤

TA-DA!

Create a good-for-you and tasty meal in a hurry.

Combine a low-calorie, low-fat, frozen chicken and pasta entrée with frozen mixed vegetables and a small can of diced tomatoes,

and voilà—delicious dinner—on the table fast! ❤

Split Thinking

INSTEAD OF A FULL-BLOWN, ALL-OUT, NO-HOLDS-BARRED, BANANA SPLIT, create your own healthy replacement. Split a banana, add a scoop of non-fat frozen yogurt, drizzle one tablespoon of chocolate syrup over it, and top with non-fat whipped cream. You can add strawberries, blueberries, or blackberries, if you like. ❤

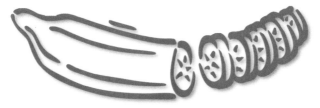

MAKING a Mockery

Whip up some mock whipped cream.

Simply keep a can of evaporated skim milk in the refrigerator. About an hour before serving, put a bowl and beaters in the freezer. When ready to serve, pour the milk into the chilled bowl, add one teaspoon of pure vanilla extract, (one teaspoon of brandy, optional), and mix at high-speed—just until soft peaks form. Spoon over fruit, pudding, or sponge cake. Finally—Enjoy! ❤

Chip OFF the Old BLOCK

By switching to mini-chocolate chips in a cookie recipe instead of the standard size,

you can save about one-half cup and 15 grams of fat and not even notice the difference. ❤

400

THICK and THIN

Instead of milk or cream to thicken soups, try purees made from vegetables. Chop the vegetable selection up in a food processor, throw in a dash of spice and add to your favorite "thick" soup recipes in place of the dairy. ❤

401

spread it out

Add strawberries, blueberries, blackberries, or other favorite fruits, to a little low-fat yogurt. Mix well. This flavorful spread is excellent on English muffins or bagels. ❤

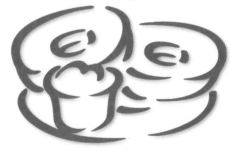

CHECk *the* LaBELS

A six-ounce can of tuna **packed in water has about two grams of fat and 160 calories;** while the same size **packed in oil has 15 grams of fat and 285 calories**—and that is after you have drained it! After you have tried a couple of the cans of the water-packed variety, you will not miss the oilier one. **PR◌MiSe!** ♥

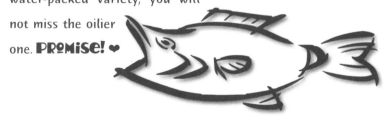

Armed with quick wit, years of professional experience, and more get-pretty tips than a beauty pageant coordinator, spa owner, expert makeup artist, esthetician, and author, Susie Galvez is dedicated to giving women tools to help them accept themselves and realize that each day is another chance to be beautiful.

Having lost over 100 pounds herself, Susie has walked the walk of a dieter, and continues to "tow the line" each and every day. Inspired by the thrill she gets from helping women rediscover beauty on a daily basis, Susie wrote *Weight Loss Wisdom: 365 successful dieting tips* to help women feel good about their appearance.

Susie is also the author of the *Ooh La La! Effortless Beauty* series which includes *Ooh La La! Perfect Face; Ooh La La! Perfect Body; Ooh La La! Perfect Makeup;*

and *Ooh La La! Perfect Hair*. She also wrote *Hello Beautiful: 365 ways to be even more beautiful*, and *InSPArations: Ideas, tips, and techniques to increase employee loyalty, client satisfaction, and bottom line spa profits*.

In addition to writing, Susie owns Face Works Day Spa in Richmond, Virginia which has been featured in magazines such as *Allure*, *Cosmopolitan*, *Elle*, and *Town and Country* as well as many trade publications including *Skin, Inc.*, *Dermascope*, *Day Spa*, *Salon Today*, *Nails Plus*, *Nails*, *Spa Management*, and *Les Nouvelles Esthetiques*.

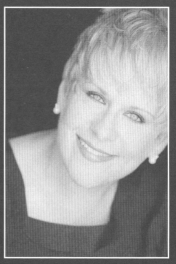

(continued)

405

Susie is also recognized as one of the leading consultants in the spa industry. She is a featured spokesperson for the beauty industry in magazines, on radio and television programs internationally and is also a member of Cosmetic Executive Women, The National Association of Women Business Owners, and the Society of American Cosmetic Chemists.

You can contact Susie at **www.susiegalvez.com** or at **www.beautyatourfingertips.com** where you will find even more ways to keep yourself looking beautiful. Be sure to sign up for your free spa-at-home tips! ❤

"Appreciation is a wonderful thing:
it makes what is excellent in others belong to us as well."
Voltaire

This book could not have been completed without the unwavering support and love from my very special friends. Thank you to:

Jody Allen, doctoral candidate, whose command of the English language and proofreading skills were once again put to the test with this mansucript, but who was always gentle in how she suggested "perhaps a better way to say it." And she, of course, was right.

Dennis Michael Stredney, graphic designer, who once again "got it" and turned my words into art.

Zaro Weil, publisher, who continues to be a friend from first sight. Thanks again for making my vision a reality.

Anne Szamboti, Cathy Cassidy, and Melissa Lane, for all the years, tears, and laughter, in fighting the weight-loss dragon.

To Amber Ensign and the wonderful staff at Face Works Day Spa who inspire me daily.

And lastly, but always first with me, thank you Tino Galvez—you are truly the wind beneath my wings. XOXO

407